3D Printing in Medicine

Contents

Introduction

Gerald T. Grant and Frank J. Rybicki

We are in the midst of a technological revolution in customized patient care. Advances in imaging techniques with digital 3D and 4D rendering and advances of 3D printing have allowed healthcare professionals the ability to view and document hard and soft tissues in such a manner that meaningful, accurate measurements can be used for fabrication of medical models for presurgical planning/patient education, fabrication of surgical templates, and medical/dental devices for implantation or quality of life. In addition, 3D print technologies in printing biological tissues will provide a future for many patients with the eventual printing of human organs.

The media continues to highlight the impact of 3D printing on patient care on local and national newscasts, and many have taken a social media approach to publicize the impact on this new, innovative way to deliver medical data. However, until recently, a single healthcare organization leader has not emerged as a home to release technologies, to disseminate the peer review literature, to manage the roles and future responsibilities of 3D printing in education, and

G.T. Grant, D.M.D., M.S.
Department of Oral Health and Rehabilitation,
University of Louisville, School of Dentistry,
Louisville, KY, USA
e-mail: gerald.grant@louisville.edu

F.J. Rybicki, M.D., Ph.D. (✉)
Department of Radiology, The University of Ottawa
Faculty of Medicine and The Ottawa Hospital
Research Institute, Ottawa, ON, Canada
e-mail: frybicki@toh.ca

to lead discussions with regulatory bodies geared for reimbursement. This, in turn, has left much of the responsibilities of current development and direction to the manufacturers, in response to individual medical and dental requests.

At the forefront of this entire process is medical imaging and dental imaging, as radiology and applied imaging science professionals largely manage the studies that identify patient-specific anatomical areas of interest for design and fabrication of customized models, surgical guides, and medical devices that are 3D printed. Moreover, much of 3D printing is from medical images, and several of the more complex steps, where errors can be introduced, are in image post-processing. This has historically been performed in radiology departments, using customized software packages and expertise inclusive in the training to become a radiologist. For this reason, radiologists feel that much is "at stake" with medical 3D printing, with enormous opportunities in the field that are tempered with the fear that "if we don't do it, someone else will...." Radiology has, in turn, stepped up to the plate. The Radiological Society of North America (RSNA) recently created its first ever "Special Interest Group," focused on 3D printing. In addition, the Journal of *3D Printing in Medicine* was recently launched and is enjoying increasing success as a resource for the peer-reviewed literature.

This book, edited by a senior dentist/prosthodontist with over 20 years of experience in 3D

F.J. Rybicki, G.T. Grant (eds.), *3D Printing in Medicine*, DOI 10.1007/978-3-319-61924-8_1

printing and an academic radiologist with 7 years' experience, is intended to introduce the field with straightforward language that will be consumable for a large audience. This book is not a comprehensive survey of all 3D printing in medicine. Moreover, bioprinting is not covered in these pages. However, the book explains 3D printing fundamentals and will serve as a highly useful reference guide to keep handy in the interpretation of the increasing body of knowledge in the literature. Dedicated chapters that focus on hardware and software applications should prove indispensable for those who are eager to enter the field. The book also has important chapters in starting a laboratory within a medical facility and the key factors in quality and safety that are an essential part of a 3D printing organization. We include authorship from close allies at the FDA who, like us, share a great interest in stewarding 3D printing from its current niche applications to more widespread use in the medical community. The book extends to include chapters on some of those niche applications. At this point in the exponential growth of 3D printing, assembling a chapter on each organ system is challenging, since the field changes dramatically between the time of writing and the date of publication. However, we have included several representative chapters so that the readership can be enriched with many examples of how 3D printing is positively influencing medicine.

1.1 History of 3D Printing in Medicine

In the mid-1990s, groups from Canada, Wales, German, and the United States (USA) as well as the US military began to experiment with the use of 3D printing for head and neck reconstruction. as a collaborative organization known as the Advanced Digital Technologies Foundation (www.adtfoundation.com). With the help of the software company Materialise (Leuven, Belgium), they were able to convert DICOM images into a Standard Tessellation Language (STL) file to 3D print. Early images were of bones, for example, the skull, and these models changed the fabrication techniques for cranial implants.

In the mid-1990s, Medical Modeling of Golden Colorado under the leadership of Andy Christensen offered a commercial service for medical models, surgical guides, and customized devices used by both healthcare professionals and the commercial medical industry. They became one of the leading groups in making this technology accessible to healthcare providers worldwide. Mr. Christensen sold the business to 3D Systems in 2014 at which point it became a pillar of 3D Systems new healthcare vertical.

In 2005, the Institute for Reconstructive Sciences in Medicine (iRSM), as part of the Alberta Health Services, Universtity of Alberta, Edmonton, Canada, developed a virtual simulation and 3D print lab. Under the direction of Dr. Johan Wolfaardt (a prosthodontist), the lab offers virtual surgical simulation, guide design and fabrication using digital techologies and 3D printing in support of head and neck reconstruction. The facility has designers, engineers, and a varity of priniting capabilites. They have been one of the international leaders in this technology along with similar facilities in Wales and Germany.

The Mayo Clinic, Rochester, MN, USA, led by Jane Matsumoto and Jonathan (Jay) Morris, was to our knowledge the first group to organize a 3D printing laboratory within a radiology department outside of the US military in the United States, and their lab has been one of the leaders in the field since. They have pioneered the production of in-house, physician-managed 3D printing within radiology, and they have the most experience globally with providing medical models, from physicians to physicians, for presurgical evaluations, patient education, and medical education, outside the US military. Drs. Matsumoto and Morris are also leading educators in the field, with extensive continuing professional development courses hosted by the Mayo Clinic.

1.2 History of 3D Printing in the US Military Medical Community

A great example of 3D printing's power is how the military leveraged the technology in its infancy and contributed greatly to its current uses. Routine use of digital planning and fabrication of medical models for the military began in the mid-1990s when Capt. Charlie Richardson, DC, USN, designed and fabricated medical models working with the Radiology Department at the National Naval Medical Center (NNMC), Bethesda, MD, USA. Medical models were fabricated of craniofacial and orthopedic bony structures that required extending manufacturing by 3 or 4 days, depending upon the model, using fused deposition modeling technologies. However, through his efforts, it was realized that computed tomography (CT) scans could provide the information needed to provide three-dimensional presurgical data. By the late 1990s, the Maxillofacial Prosthetics Department at the Naval Postgraduate Dental School (NPDS) began to apply this technology to fabricate cranial implants. A model of the skull was used to sculpt a cranial plate from wax, a mold was developed, and a polymethylmethacrylate (PMMA) implant was processed. The result was a well-fitting implant requiring little to no adjustments, with a concurrent 50% reduction in operating room time. However, the fabrication process was still time-consuming. By early 2000, stereolithography (SLA) additive manufacturing technology became available at the Walter Reed Army Medical Center (WRAMC) under contract to Stephen Rouse, DDS (retired USA), shortening the model fabrication time. This launched fabrication, not only for models in support of cranial implants with NPDS but in support of orthopedics and neurosurgery. The direction of the development and use of this technology became paramount for reconstruction and rehabilitation of wounded warriors with the beginning of the war on terrorism in late 2001. The collaboration of the WRAMC and NPDS team became essential, in that they were able to pioneer many different techniques to fabricate cranial implants and cutting guides that provided unprecedented care in wounded warrior craniotomy/cranioplasty, and by 2005 the residual calvarial bone from the osteotomy that was usually saved for reimplantation was no longer used.

While design software techniques worked well when one could "mirror" a non-affected (presumed to be normal) side, solutions for midface defects were more difficult to develop. In 2007, Capt Gerald Grant DC, USN, was awarded funding to develop a method to capture pre-combat craniofacial records. This resulted in the introduction of dental cone beam computed tomography (CBCT) technologies to the Department of Defense as well as 3D photographic technologies of the individual that could be registered to the CBCT. They were able to put together a team, NPDS Craniofacial Imaging Research, that began to work closely with WRAMC and develop techniques for registration, surgical guide fabrication, and implant designs. A SLA device and design software's were purchased and installed at NPDS, and the development of presurgical teams was introduced to NNMC and WRAMC in craniofacial reconstructions to neurosurgery, oral maxillofacial surgery, otolaryngology, orthopedic surgery, and plastic surgery. From this laboratory, several relationships were formed, including one with academic medical centers such as John's Hopkins Hospital, Baltimore, MD, and the Brigham and Women's Hospital, in Boston, MA, USA. It was in this capacity that Dr. Frank Rybicki began collaborating as part of the face transplantation program led by the innovative and brilliant surgeon Bohdan Pomahac, MD.

The BRAC (Defense Base and Realignment and Closure) initiative provided an opportunity to combine the assets at WRAMC with those at NPDS, and a site was selected that co-located the facilities to provide better collaboration with the BRAC assets co-located with the Maxillofacial Prosthetics Laboratory. The new 3D Medical Applications Center (3DMAC) fell under the Department of Radiology at Walter Reed National Military Medical Center Bethesda (WRNMMCB), and the services were expanded to include many different additive manufacturing systems, such as titanium which allowed direct fabrication of cranial implants, and access was expanded worldwide via a public secured website. This expanded the use of these technologies to orthopedics, pediatrics, ophthalmology, limb prosthetics, occupational health, maxillofacial prostheses, dental, and a host of research activities worldwide. The staff was expanded to include a PhD biomedical engineer, a metals engineer, and two CT technicians to design anatomical models that worked in conjunction with NPDS's craniofacial imaging team, which included an aerospace engineer, two staff maxillofacial prosthodontists, rotating residents, and rotating midshipmen from the United States Naval Academy as part of the Capstone Program to increase development of advanced medical/digital technologies in treatment of wounded warriors.

3D printing continues to be used for customized patient-specific treatments at WRNMMCB. Custom fabricated cranial and reconstruction titanium implants are fabricated for patient-specific implantation. Presurgical medical models, medical devices, and custom attachments for prosthetic limbs have been developed to accommodate wounded warriors to improve surgical outcomes, quality of life, assist in medical research, and provide customizable devices for occupational health.

1.3   Current 3D Printing

Medical 3D printing centers span both industry and civilian medical centers. There are several service models to obtain printed models, including outsource images (e.g., a CT scan or MR images) to vendors such as Materialise who in turn provide consultation and 3D printing. Similarly, recent years have seen collaboration between software and hardware companies, for example, Vital Images and Stratasys, two leaders in their respective fields of 3D visualization and 3D printing hardware, have marketed a service model designed to leverage expertise from both sides to accept auto segmented STL files and provide models.

Many medical centers have begun to emulate the organization and infrastructure from the Mayo Clinic, capitalizing on the medical expertise in house and assembling the physical and human resources needed for a functioning lab. These are detailed in a chapter in this book, based on the laboratory at the University of Ottawa Faculty of Medicine. Education has provided a bridge to other centers. Beginning in 2013, the RSNA has hosted didactic sessions in 3D printing, and for the past several years, hands-on courses have been available, with the number of students in these teaching sessions exceeding 1000.

To meet the needs of medical 3D printing, the manufacturers such as 3D Systems and Stratasys have begun to develop printers that provide the ability to print open vessels, different colors, and a variety of materials. For more than a dozen years, the medical sector has been featured at the Society of Mechanical Engineers (SME) RAPID meeting. Finally, workgroups within the SME have begun to engage with the community, in particular to work, as other groups have, to look at medical reimbursement. Comments on these important discussions are also covered in later chapters.

3D printing is truly one of the leading technologies of our time; we hope that this book will provide essential information and that it will help you understand the impact that 3D printing can have on medicine in the hopes of improving the outcomes and quality of life for many patients around the world. Finally, we genuinely believe that the leaders in the next generation of 3D printing will be reading this book and that we can inspire others to enter the field and make gainful contributions.

3D Printing Technologies

2

Dimitrios Mitsouras and Peter C. Liacouras

2.1 Introduction

The first three-dimensional (3D) printing technology was invented in the early 1980s to fill the need for rapid engineering of design prototypes. The process, also known as "rapid prototyping" and "additive manufacturing," widely expanded in the fields of architecture and manufacturing in the 1990s. Today there is a multitude of diverse 3D printing technologies that can manufacture objects using a vast array of materials, from thermoplastics and polymers to metal, capable of fulfilling most engineering and design needs. Medical applications of 3D printing can be tracked to the mid-1990s. It is only within the last 5 years, that it has gained tremendous momentum and is now used daily in hospitals and private practices around the globe.

An early "3D printing lab" is rapidly emerging in many medical specialties. Many of these labs are in academic hospital radiology departments, while others are in cardiac or orthopedic surgery departments and practices. Their development will likely mirror the path of the "3D lab" as it evolved in radiology departments around the world. 3D labs began emerging more than a decade ago to fill the need of radiologists to communicate pertinent findings to medical care teams by visualizing the 3D volumetric imaging data acquired by diverse medical imaging modalities in anatomic rather than traditional acquisition planes (Fishman et al. 1987; Rubin et al. 1993). A handheld model derived from DICOM images represents a natural progression from its 3D visualization. The demand for such "anatomic" 3D-printed models for interventional planning is poised to grow as the technology becomes more available (Mitsouras et al. 2015; Giannopoulos et al. 2016). However, 3D printers offer a multitude of opportunities to benefit medical practice beyond anatomic visualization and hands-on surgical simulation. With 3D printing, patient-specific implants, guides, prosthetics, molds, and tools can also be manufactured to directly treat patients. This creates opportunities for 3D printing centers to be housed in hospital departments, for example, prosthetics, where the corresponding expertise exists. However, due to the large investment, it is economically sensible for hospitals to avoid duplicating these centers across specialties, and thus the model emerging in some

D. Mitsouras, Ph.D. (✉)
Applied Imaging Science Lab, Department of Radiology, Brigham and Women's Hospital, Harvard Medical School, Boston, MA, USA

Department of Biochemistry Microbiology and Immunology, The University of Ottawa, Faculty of Medicine, Ottawa, ON, Canada
e-mail: dmitsouras@alum.mit.edu

P.C. Liacouras, Ph.D.
3D Medical Applications Center, Department of Radiology, Walter Reed National Military Medical Center (WRNMMC), Bldg 1, Rm 4417B, 8901 Wisconsin Avenue, Bethesda, MD 20889, USA
e-mail: peter.c.liacouras.civ@mail.mil

© Springer International Publishing AG 2017
F.J. Rybicki, G.T. Grant (eds.), *3D Printing in Medicine*, DOI 10.1007/978-3-319-61924-8_2

institutions at the forefront of the technology involves a single 3D lab that is in its own division, staffed with faculty across specialties and cross appointed to that division. Such a centralized 3D printing division can effectively serve the needs of an entire hospital.

Until the technology is sufficiently proven and high-quantity "production" parts become commonplace in medical practice to support such centralized processes, rapid implementation of the 3D printing lab is currently underway in radiology, empowered by decreasing 3D printing costs and improvements in software tools to convert DICOM images to 3D-printed objects. The substantial start-up financial and physical space costs of purchasing and operating a 3D printer need to be wisely invested based on the needs of each practice. Furthermore, there are many factors which contribute to the construction of an accurate 3D-printed model (George et al. 2017a). Doing so requires diverse staff that possess expertise spanning many disciplines from engineering, physics, chemistry, to medical specialties starting with radiology and surgical and rehabilitation specialties. This chapter reviews 3D printing technologies without assuming a specific background so that all stakeholders may utilize it. The review of 3D printer capabilities, including communicating 3D models to them and the types of materials they can use, will assist the clinical practice in the informed investment of a 3D printing technology based on specific clinical needs.

The first additive manufacturing technology, stereolithography (SLA), was invented in 1980, patented in 1983, and commercialized by 3D Systems in 1987. Many other 3D printing technologies have since emerged that use energy or chemistry to produce printed objects. At present, the term 3D printing is used to collectively refer to additive manufacturing technologies or rapid prototyping. We have prioritized the technologies used for 3D printing from medical images based on emerging uses reported in the medical literature, including pre-/postsurgical models, custom surgical guides, prosthetics, and customized 3D-printed implants. 3D printing in medicine involves the fabrication of organs depicted in

DICOM images, and potentially tools, guides, and implants that fit those organs. 3D bioprinting, the process by which living replacement tissues or organs are manufactured, is not covered in this chapter.

2.1.1 Communicating with a 3D Printer: The Standard Tessellation File Format and Beyond

3D printers cannot interpret DICOM images. Instead, 3D printing technologies accept a digital description of a 3D model, which they then manufacture into a physical object. To date, these digital object descriptions are limited to 3D surfaces that enclose a region of space. A 3D printer manufactures these objects by filling (entirely or in a porous fashion) the space enclosed by each such surface with a solid material. The solid material is created by energy deposition, for example, by melting a solid and selectively laying it in the region enclosed by that surface, or by a chemical reaction, for example, by solidifying a liquid selectively in the locations enclosed by that surface. How these surfaces are described and stored is thus a critical component of understanding and using 3D printing technologies. How these surfaces are generated from a patient's DICOM images to describe the specific organ, tool, guide, or implant that is to be manufactured is discussed in Chap. 3.

A standard file format to define these surfaces is the Standard Tessellation Language or, as also commonly referred to, the stereolithography file format, abbreviated as "STL." The STL format defines surfaces as a collection of triangles (called facets) that perfectly fit together without any gaps, like a jigsaw puzzle (Fig. 2.1). There are two types of STL files: "binary" STL files that can only describe a single "part" and "ASCII" STL files that can contain multiple independent parts. A single part is a single, fully connected surface that encloses a single region of space. It can be printed with a single material property (e.g., a specific color and hardness). STL files are thus ideal for printing a single organ, implant, guide, or

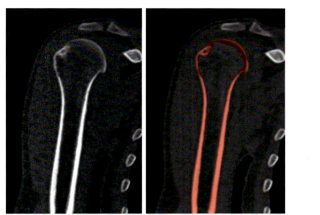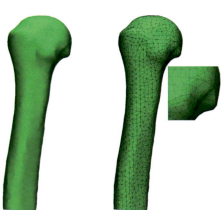

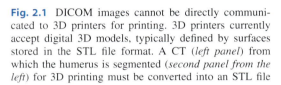

Fig. 2.1 DICOM images cannot be directly communicated to 3D printers for printing. 3D printers currently accept digital 3D models, typically defined by surfaces stored in the STL file format. A CT (*left panel*) from which the humerus is segmented (*second panel from the left*) for 3D printing must be converted into an STL file (*two right-most panels*) for sending to the 3D printer. Although STL files are usually presented by a rendering (*third panel from the right*), the underlying surface is in fact composed of simple triangles (*far right panel*) that fit together precisely and exactly as a jigsaw puzzle, with no gaps between any triangles (*inset*)

component of a tool that is not connected to other components (e.g., a single gear of a tool). This is a limiting format for medical printing. For example, if one wishes to 3D print a vessel wall with a calcified deposit, with the wall and calcification printed in different color and/or with different material properties (e.g., a soft material for the wall and a hard material for the calcification), two STL surfaces are required, and these must be stored in either two binary STL files, one for the vessel wall, and one for the calcification, or one ASCII STL file. Some printers restrict printing all objects in a single ASCII file with a single material, so that the latter is not an option.

In any case, the operator generating these STL files must not only ensure that the tissues described in the files accurately represent the anatomy, but also that the two models touch along a single side of each of the two surfaces described by the STL files, without leaving any space between them, otherwise the printed model would neither reflect physiology nor remain in one piece after printing. This approach does not scale well; for example, there is no simple way to use STL files to print this vessel if it contains a mixed plaque, with several small calcifications within a lipid-rich core. For this example, a digital description of the plaque model would ideally describe a single ana-

tomic model (plaque) and differentiate only specific locations within that model that are calcified versus lipid-rich so that they can be printed with different materials of, e.g., different colors to reflect their different tissue properties, rather than requiring independent STL files for each small calcification. Furthermore, STL files offer no opportunity to manufacture an object with a graded transition between two or more 3D printing materials, which could be used to 3D print a model that also conveys tissue "texture." For example, it is not readily possible to print cancellous bone with inhomogeneous material properties (e.g., hardness) that could represent information regarding trabeculae and marrow or the gradual transition to healthy tissue in the case of an infiltrating tumor.

Approaches to achieve 3D printing of organs with inhomogeneous material properties are an active area of research to enable medical models to convey not only tissue biomechanical properties but also radiographic properties. For example, we are actively exploring the use of inhomogeneous 3D printing material mixtures when printing a single organ to be able to generate a printed model that replicates the image signal characteristics of the organ under computed tomography (CT) and magnetic resonance

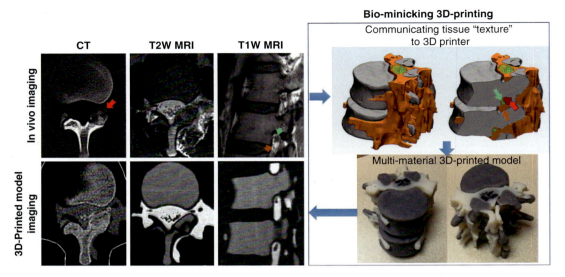

Fig. 2.2 3D-printed model of a patient with L1 left lamina osteoblastoma that replicates radiographic signal intensities similarly to in vivo patient imaging, including the tumor (*red arrows*), adipose tissue including foraminal fat (*brown arrows*), and spinal nerves (*green arrows*). At present there is no way to readily communicate such models to 3D printers

(MR) imaging (George et al. 2017b; Mitsouras et al. 2017; Guenette et al. 2016; Mayer et al. 2015). Such radiographically "biomimicking" models (Fig. 2.2) could enable the use of 3D printing for interventional radiology procedures such as thermal and nonthermal ablations, ultrasound-guided biopsies, and invasive catheter angiography-based procedures that are an important field in which 3D printing currently has only limited applications.

A second limitation of STL files is that there is no standard that is portable across softwares to store the intended color and material properties for a tissue model. At present, 3D printer-specific software is used to assign these properties to each STL file loaded for printing, which can be a tedious process and error-prone if there is a disconnect between the needs of the clinician producing the model and the technician running the printer.

The Additive Manufacturing File Format (AMF) and 3D Manufacturing Format (3MF) are newer file formats designed to overcome many of the limitations of the simple STL format, including the ability to incorporate features such as surface texture, color, and material properties into each part (Hiller and Lipson 2009). The AMF

format standard was approved by the American Society of Testing and Materials (ASTM) in June 2011 (ISO/ASTM 2016), but with a few exceptions, it is not yet available in most softwares used to convert DICOM images into 3D-printable models. We expect it will become more commonplace in the next few years as the medical applications of 3D printing are expanded to better fit the richness of tissues differentiated by present-day imaging, for example, producing elastic vascular models with embedded hard plastics to represent stents or calcifications.

It is likely however that these newer formats will also be insufficient for emerging specialized medical applications, for example, the interventional radiology paradigm described above, where each location in the interior of a digital organ model would ideally need to be assigned different material properties (e.g., to achieve a model that possesses different CT numbers or MR signal intensities within the 3D-printed volume). We expect such complex medical 3D applications will lead to the development of additional file formats that are less reliant on the concept of a set of solid "parts" (e.g., organs) each of which has a single set of color and material properties. Such future file formats will likely enable one to specify, radiologic and/or mechanical material properties within the volume occupied by the tissue to be printed, corresponding more directly to the concept of an organ composed of multiple tissues rather than a "part" commonly considered in engineering 3D printing applications.

2.1.2 3D Printing Technologies

3D printers use data encoded in the STL, AMF or other file format to successively fuse or deposit thin layers of material. Each layer is circumscribed by a set of closed curves that trace the outer surface(s) of the object being manufactured at that corresponding layer. The printer manufactures each such layer by filling the area enclosed by those curves with a material at a specified thickness (e.g., 0.1 mm). This is similar to the process of segmenting a tissue by successively identifying 2D regions of interest (ROIs) that circumscribe the tissue on consecutive cross-sectional images, each of which was acquired at a given fixed slice thickness. The 2D ROI is considered to fully circumscribe the tissue (and only that tissue) throughout the entire thickness of that cross section.

The taxonomy and terminology of 3D printing, which conveys how each printer's technology achieves the process of solidifying each layer and/or the fusion of the successive layers, are rapidly evolving. Complicating matters further, to date there has been no standardization of the nomenclature used in the biomedical literature to convey these different processes (Chepelev et al. 2017). However, a thorough understanding of the principles of each technology using a current, commonly accepted classification (Huang and Leu 2013) adopted as ASTM standard F2792 and International Organization for Standardization (ISO) standard 17296-2:2015 (ISO 2015) enables the end user to understand, interpret, and replicate the various techniques published in the literature.

In the current standards classifications, there are seven specific groups of technologies. These are vat photopolymerization, material jetting, binder jetting, material extrusion, powder bed fusion, sheet lamination, and directed energy deposition. The first five technologies are those most commonly encountered in medicine. Sheet lamination and directed energy deposition are less commonly utilized but still may provide a benefit when used for certain applications. Each technology has strengths and weaknesses as it pertains to its uses in clinical 3D printing (Table 2.1), and these are reviewed below.

2.1.2.1 Vat Photopolymerization

This 3D printing process is more widely known as stereolithography (SLA) or Digital Light Processing (DLP). It has three basic components: first, a high intensity light source (typically ultraviolet [UV]-A or UV-B); second, a vat or tray that holds an epoxy- or acrylic-based photo-curable liquid resin which contains monomers and oligomers; and third, a controlling system that directs the light source to selectively illuminate the resin (see below). Layers of the resin are sequentially cured by exposing it to the light source in the shape of only that cross section (i.e., ROI) of the model that is being built at that layer (perpendicular to the printer's z-axis). The light initiates a chemical reaction in the resin which causes the monomers and oligomers to polymerize and become solid. Once a layer of the object becomes structurally stable, the model is lowered (or raised, for bottom-up printers) by one layer thickness away from the active layer so that liquid resin now covers the top (or the bottom for bottom-up printers) of the previously printed layer. Polymerization of each layer is typically not fully completed by the controlled light source in order to allow the next layer to bond to the last one.

Each layer thickness is thus printed until the final layer is complete. After printing, excess resin is drained, and a solvent or alcohol rinse (generally in an industrial parts washer) is used to clean the model. Lattice support structures (Fig. 2.3) that are automatically added by the printer to achieve printing of overhangs also need to be manually removed. A final post-processing step is required, which involves "curing" the model in a UV chamber to complete polymerization of the

Table 2.1 Summary of characteristics of 3D printing technologies commonly encountered in medicine, professional equipment (>$5000) only

Technology	Other common technology names	Common material(s)	Accuracy	Cost	Advantages (generally)	Disadvantages (generally)
Vat photopolymerization	Stereolithography (SLA) Digital light processing (DLP) Continuous digital light processing (CLIP)	Epoxy- and acrylic-based polymers Infused polymers	+++	$$	Accuracy Biocompatible (short-term) materials available Can print small hollow vessels with no intraluminal support Microprinting possible (e.g., for microfluidics)	Brittle, moderate strength Models are single material Limited color options
Material jetting	MultiJet Printing (MJP) Polyjet	Acrylic-based polymers	+++	$$	Accuracy, variety of materials Models can be multi-material/multicolor Biocompatible (short-term) materials available	Moderate strength
Material extrusion	Fused deposition modeling (FDM)	ABS, PLA plastics, composites, metals (rare)	+	$	Low cost Strong, durable materials	Lower accuracy Model surfaces have prominent stair stepping ridges
Binder jetting		Gypsum, sand, metal (rare)	+	$	Speed Variety of materials Color capability in external shell No attached supports	Low strength Model infiltration is necessary
Powder bed fusion	Electron beam melting (EBM) Selective laser sintering (SLS) Direct metal laser sintering (DMLS) Selective laser melting (SLM) MultiJet Fusion (MJF)	Plastics, synthetic polymers, metal	++	$$$	Diverse mechanical properties Variety of materials Material strength sufficient for functional parts Long-term biocompatible (implantable) materials available Attached supports not usually required (nonmetals)	Various finishes (dependent on the machine) Models are single material

Note: This table is a generalization of the multiple technologies; some exceptions will exist

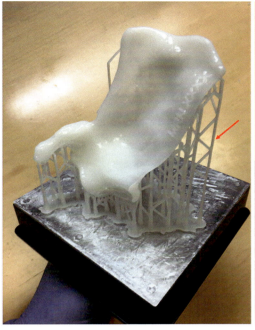
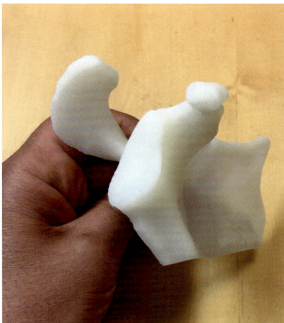

Fig. 2.3 Example of model of a scapula 3D printed using a bottom-up stereolithography vat photopolymerization 3D printer. During printing, the printer also prints a lattice of support rods (*red arrow*) that allow printing those portions of the model that would otherwise have nothing underneath them to support the printed material

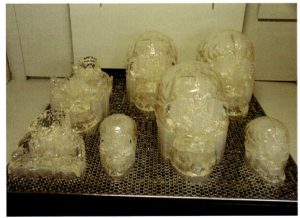
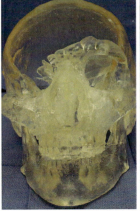
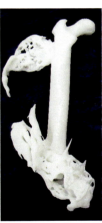

Fig. 2.4 Models 3D printed using a large, professional top-to-bottom stereolithography vat photopolymerization 3D printer (*left panel*). Printed models need to undergo UV curing to finish. Lattice supports present must be removed during model post-processing. Materials and machine size can vary

layer bonds (Fig. 2.4), rendering this as one of the more labor-intensive methods. Finishing may also be required, for example, to smooth step edges (light sanding) and application of a UV-resistant sealant.

The difference between SLA and DLP is the light source and how it is controlled to selectively illuminate and cure the resin. In SLA, the light source is a laser which is directed by mirrors to different locations on the liquid's surface (x–y

plane). The mirrors continuously and progressively cause the laser to trace the entire area of each layer of the object being printed. DLP instead uses a projector, such as those used in movie theaters, which instantly illuminates the entire shape of the layer of the object being printed onto the liquid's surface. DLP tends to require less time to print an object as each layer doesn't need to be progressively "raster scanned" but, apart from specific machines, most often lacks the high resolution of SLA afforded by a laser beam. An exciting new bottom-up DLP printer technology has been recently developed that uses an oxygen-inhibiting layer or "dead zone" above a membrane that sits at the bottom of the vat holding the resin. The oxygen layer inhibits polymerization at the interface of the membrane and the printed object. This proprietary technique, termed "continuous liquid interface production" (CLIP) by one 3D printer manufacturer (Carbon 3D, Redwood City, CA), reduces the mechanical steps involved in vat photopolymerization, offering prints at one or two orders of magnitude faster than other 3D printing technologies (Tumbleston et al. 2015), and can be as short as 5–10 min for, e.g., a scapula. Other similar approaches such as the Intelligent Liquid Interface (ILI™, NewPro3D, Vancouver, Canada) can provide larger build platforms, drastically cutting down build speeds and limitations on size. Mechanical steps are otherwise required in bottom-up printers to free the last printed layer from the transparent material (e.g., glass) floor of the vat to which the polymer adheres to as a consequence of the polymerization process. These steps typically involve lowering or shifting the vat by a small amount until the model, held in place by a base at the top, has come fully loose from the vat floor and subsequently returning the vat to just one layer thickness away from the previously printed layer. This process, in conjunction with constraints placed by the resin, e.g., to relieve internal stresses between layers and to allow flow of new resin below the model, accounts for the bulk of printing time with this technology.

Vat photopolymerization is frequently used for medical 3D printing, particularly for bone applications. It is also the only technology with which it is possible (with sufficient care taken in orienting the model in the build tray) to print hollow vessel lumens that are not filled with solid support material (Fig. 2.5) that may pose significant difficulty in removing, particularly for small, long, or tortuous vessels such as the coronaries, cerebrovasculature, and visceral aortic branches. However, materials are relatively expensive ~$210/kg. Top-down SLA printers require the resin to be maintained at a specific level in the vat, which can involve a costly investment for printers with larger build envelopes. Generally, the widely used commercial machine's build platform sizes range from less than 12.5 × 12.5 × 12.5 cm to as large as 210 × 70 × 80 cm or more. The smaller, desktop devices are often used to fabricate dental models and implant guides and hearing aids. Photopolymer materials are available in many colors and opacities ranging to translucent, as well as with material mechanical properties, such as flexible or rigid (Fig. 2.5). Older stereolithography-printed parts were relatively fragile. Newer acrylonitrile butadiene styrene (ABS)-"like" materials offer improved mechanical properties. Finally, short-term biocompatible material (see Sect. 2.2 below) are available and can be used to print sterilizable surgical tools and guides with appropriate post-processing. It is recommended to follow the manufacturer's specifications for proper material post-processing, cleaning, and sterilization particularly, but not only for tools and guides.

It is important to note that commercially available vat photopolymerization can print a model containing only a single material (color/properties), as only one liquid resin can be held in the machine's vat. To produce medical models with multiple materials (e.g., colors), each part of the model needs to be separately printed and later assembled together (Fig. 2.6). Transparent materials exist for higher-end printers that allow highlighting of internal structures (such as nerve spaces, tumors, teeth, plates) in the printed anatomy. This is done in the printer software by overexposing the material in the precise anatomical regions of those internal structures. The highlighting occurs via overexposure of the resin to the light source, that can be achieved e.g.,

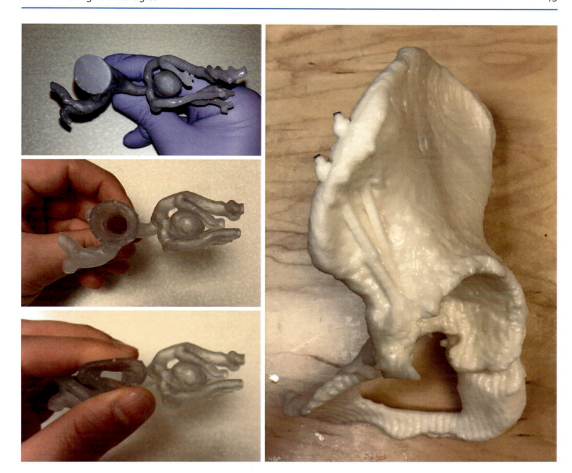

Fig. 2.5 Applications for which vat photopolymerization 3D printer technology is well suited, namely, small arterial models and particularly hollow models printed with a flexible material where a support lattice is only required external to the lumen with appropriate positioning of the model on the build tray (renal artery aneurysm shown in the *left hand panel*) and bone 3D printing (hemipelvis with prior hardware in the *right panel*)

by adding multiple copies of the structures to be highlighted (leading to multiple exposures of those model regions), or slowing the laser speed or increasing the laser intensity when printing those regions. The additional energy in this step tints the resin or activates a color additive within the resin to create the contrast. Finally, depending on the desired physical and mechanical properties of the photopolymer material, a heat treatment of 4 or more hours may be required. Thus, vat photopolymerization produces some of the smoothest, high-resolution models among 3D printing technologies, although it has limited versatility for printing multicolor/material models. In most cases, the lengthier (rate-limiting)

step is the printing itself. New CLIP and ILI™ technologies can offer extremely fast printing speeds compared to other technologies, but cleaning and post-processing procedures may then become the rate-limiting step.

2.1.2.2 Material Jetting

Material jetting is a different technology but related to vat photopolymerization in that it relies on the same chemical principles. Unlike vat photopolymerization printers, material jetting printers do not hold the material in a vat. Instead, they are analogous to inkjet document printers. Just as inkjet printers jet ink onto paper and allow it to dry, material jetting 3D printers jet microdroplets

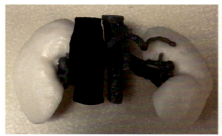
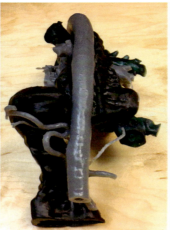
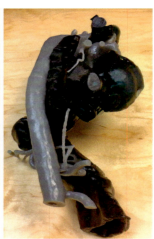

Fig. 2.6 Example of model of a bilateral renal aneurysm printed with vat photopolymerization (*left-hand panel*) with arteries printed in *gray*, veins in *black*, and kidneys in *white*. Each component was printed separately using the different-colored resins and later meticulously assembled together. This is not always readily (or at all) possible as shown for a model of a distal esophageal gastrointestinal stromal tumor (GIST) where the aorta curves around the esophagus (*right-hand panel*). This required printing the aorta in three pieces for assembly around the systemic veins and GI tract

of liquid photopolymer resin onto a build tray and polymerize it with UV light. The jetting heads scan across the build tray (e.g., left to right and front to back, i.e., the printer's x–y axes), and a controller instructs them to spray/extrude microdroplets of the resin only when passing above those locations that are to be filled for the layer of the part currently being printed. Once the layer is completed, the build tray is incrementally lowered, and the jetting heads begin scanning across the x–y plane to print the next layer. In some printers, the print heads rise, while in others, the build platform lowers by one layer thickness to print subsequent layers. Two or more sets of jetting heads are required, one set for the photopolymer used to build the model and one set for "support material." The support material is a gel-like or wax material necessary to support overhangs and complicated geometries. Overhang support is essential to the build success of this technology, since resin cannot be jetted onto empty space below (Fig. 2.7). The composition of the support dictates the removal process. Common support removal processes include soaking in mild soap solutions, by hand, with pressurized water sprays, or by melting. Other part post-processing such as

curing is not typically required, except for specific materials, e.g., a thermal treatment can enhance the printed part's thermal properties, to increase the part's heat deflection temperature. While like SLA material jetting enjoys high resolution, of the order of a few tens of microns in all three axes, models tend to have a matte surface finish. This may create a need to apply clear coat (paint or resin) to models to enhance transparency for clear materials and to give a smooth model appearance.

Overall, material jetting machines are a versatile technology for printing anatomic medical models. Material can more easily be swapped than for vat photo polymerization printers, since they are stored in cartridges, and multi-material machines allow for numerous different material colors and properties to be used to print a single model. Multi-material printers have multiple print heads, enabling a single model to be printed containing regions printed with each of the materials loaded in each print head. For example, transparent organ models can be easily printed with internal elements such as nerves, vessels, hardware, or tumors, each visible in a different opaque color (Fig. 2.7). In higher-end printers,

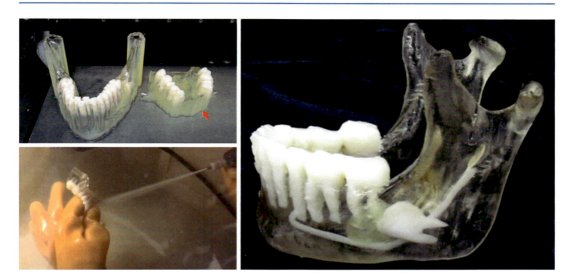

Fig. 2.7 Model of a mandible highlighting internal features (teeth, impacted molar, alveolar canal, and cyst) 3D printed using a material jetting printer. Support material (*red arrow, top left panel*) is removed using a water jet (*bottom left panel*). The model is then allowed to dry, and a clear coat is applied to aid in transparency yielding the final product (*right-hand panel*). In the above picture, one can see a mandible with internal features (teeth, impacted molar, alveolar canal, and cyst highlighted

the materials in each print head can also be mixed during the printing, thus allowing for tens to hundreds of "digital" materials (i.e., on-the-fly created combinations of materials) to be used to print a single model (Fig. 2.8). This is done by controlling the relative ratio and multiplexing of the microdroplets jetted from each head when printing each location of the object, allowing seamless mixing of the different materials held in each head. Flexible materials are also available and when mixed with a solid can be used to achieve different durometer (hardness) and mechanical properties, ranging from flexible (rubberlike) to hard/rigid. For numerous of these machines, short-term biocompatible material is available for printing of surgical tools and guides. A number of manufacturers of this technology market machines specifically for dental casts and dental implant guides. Again, it is recommended to follow the manufacturer's specifications for proper model post-processing, cleaning, and sterilization.

Material costs are among the highest across 3D printing modalities, (~$300/kg), but are delivered in cartridges for as-needed use. Each individual printer manufacturer tightly controls

materials, using microchips located within the cartridges that are read by the printer to identify the cartridge. In addition to the inability to use third-party materials, expiration dates stored on the chip block material limit use after expiration. Machines with different-size platforms are available with a maximum size of $100 \times 80 \times 50$ cm, but the technology is somewhat slow, with, for example, a pelvis requiring of the order of 24–48 h to print, rendering printing time the rate-limiting step.

2.1.2.3 Binder Jetting

Binder jet printers are also in some aspects similar to document inkjet printers. A print head scans the x–y plane and jets a liquid binding agent on to a bed of fine powder in the shape of the currently printed layer of the object. The binding agent selectively bonds the powder wherever deposited. Many binder jetting printers incorporate color print heads or binders, to achieve color either throughout or only on the outer (visible) surface of the model. Colors in a large range are possible with this technique, similar to that of paper-printed documents. The color is achieved by either mixing multiple colored binders or mixing colored ink

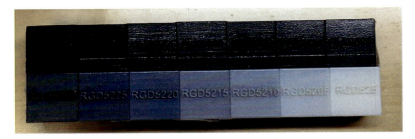

Fig. 2.8 High-end material jetting printers allow printing models using mixtures of two to four base resins loaded into the machine. Here, 14 cubes were printed in a machine with two material heads, one loaded with a flexible black-colored material (cube in *top left corner* was printed with that material at 100%) and the other loaded with a rigid white material (cube in *bottom right corner*). The cubes between these two were printed with a "digital" mixture (specially designed matrix of interwoven droplets from each material) to achieve different mixtures of the two base materials having different properties from flexible to increasingly rigid and color from black to white

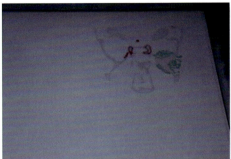 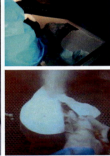 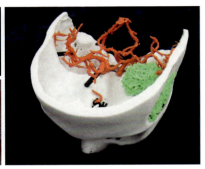

Fig. 2.9 Model of skull printed using a binder jet printer. Powder bed onto which colored binder has been laid is shown mid-print (*left panel*). Once the print is completed, the model is dug out from the powder using a vacuum (*middle panel top row*), and any unbound powder remaining is removed using an air jet (*middle panel bottom row*). The model is completed by infiltration to strengthen it (*right-hand panel*)

onto a monochrome, usually white, binder during the jetting process. After each layer is bonded, the build tray is lowered, and a roller is used to deposit a new thin layer of powder covering the print tray. Binder jet offers a versatile option for economical printing of multicolor models, with the color palette of a single model easily being in the thousands of colors. Limitations of commercial printers in this family are the inability to print translucent or flexible models and that the printed models can be composed of only a single powder, usually primarily composed of gypsum, ceramic, or sand. Printed models are rough in surface finish, and intricate models are fragile before post-processing (Fig. 2.9). Post-processing involves first vacuuming and blowing off unbonded powder to clean the model and then "infiltration" of the model with cyanoacrylate, wax, resin, or metal. The choice of infiltrate is dictated by the material in the printer and contributes to the final strength of the part. Generally, for medical models printed with powder composed primarily of gypsum, sealing with cyanoacrylate is adequate. With some materials, infiltrating with an elastomer can be used to produce models that are somewhat deformable (elastic). It is unlikely that biocompatible models can be easily produced with this technology as powders, binders, infiltrates, and possible infiltration depth would all affect biocompatibility; however, it may be possible to attain this characteristic with certain infiltration processes.

Binder jetting is used extensively to print models for anatomic visualization with color-coded anatomy (Fig. 2.9). Newer software also allows for bony anatomy to be colored according to the bone density and vascular data populated from DICOM reconstructions such as typical 3D visualizations. The popularity of this technology is driven by two significant strengths. First, materials are relatively less expensive than other printing modalities, at ~$150/kg after infiltration. Second, support structures are not needed since the model is continuously supported by unbonded powder that fills the build tray during fabrication. This allows fine overhanging structures such as small vessels to be directly printed *a proviso* great care in powder removal and model cleaning is exercised, since the plaster-like or sand materials are generally fragile before infiltration. Accordingly, care must be taken in general when recovering the printed model to ensure that small pieces are not damaged. In special cases, support structures can also be incorporated so that larger overhangs of a model will not fracture from its own weight and green strength during the powder removal process. The largest build platform currently available is roughly $180 \times 100 \times 70$ cm. This technology is widely used in medicine for anatomic models due to its affordability, reliability, and speed capable of, e.g., printing a full skull in approximately 8 h, color capability, and ability to print parts without supports attachment sites that need to be disloged (broken off) the model.

2.1.2.4 Material Extrusion

Material extrusion, also known as fused deposition modeling (FDM), represents the most widespread and economical 3D printing technology, especially when including nonmedical applications. It is the most commonly used technology for consumer-based "at home" printers and has thus been widely used by researchers in medical 3D printing. Due to the broad range of printers that fall into this category, this chapter will focus primarily on FDM 3D printers viewed as commercial machines. In this technology, one or more heated extrusion head(s) are used to melt a thermoplastic filament and deposit it selectively on the build tray in the shape of the layer of the object being printed. The extrusion heads and/or the build tray move in the x–y plane in a path precomputed by the printer driver software to efficiently trace the shape of the printed object at each layer. Once extruded at each location occu-

pied by the object, the material hardens by cooling. The material is typically a filament wound on a coil which is unreeled by motors feeding it to the extrusion head.

Various thermoplastics including ABS and polylactic acid (PLA) plastics, and polymers including biocompatible polyether ether ketone (PEEK) and metals can be printed with FDM. Biocompatible thermoplastics are available, for example, ABS that can be gamma or ethylene oxide sterilized. Specific printers tend to use materials specific to the hardware. Most "at-home" printers have a single extrusion head, allowing only a single material to be printed at a time. In these lower-end printers, supporting lattices are made of the same printing material and can be extremely difficult to pry off. Most medical models have difficultly printing with these printers, as printing the complex overhangs of human anatomic structures (e.g., visceral aortic branches) in thermoplastics will most likely deform if inappropriately supported. Most commercial-grade printers possess a second extruding head allowing a support material to be used. This support material is typically soluble in a hot water or other solvent (e.g., weak lye solution) bath; however, depending on the material one desires to print, dissolvable supports may not be available as not all materials will stick to the currently available support material. Occasionally, machines that possess additional print heads can be used to print a model that contains multiple colors and/or materials. The finish quality of FDM-printed parts is generally inferior to other technologies, due to both the fact that typical layer thickness is approximately 250 μm, larger than with other technologies, as well as because bonding at the interfaces of consecutively extruded tubular filaments is partial, with voids in the mesostructure (Fig. 2.10). However, printers are now capable of printing near 100 μm or less, similar to that of the previous technologies, offering improved finish. Nonetheless, FDM models may be suboptimal for simulation of endovascular procedures, especially when printed at larger layer thicknesses, as in addition to the rough surface

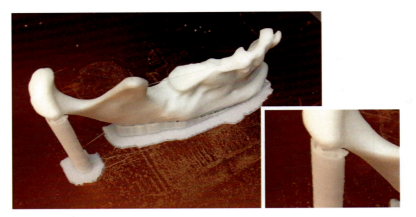

Fig. 2.10 Model of a hemimandible 3D printed using a material extrusion printer. *Inset* shows the typical striations on the surface of models printed with this technology due to its typically lower layer resolution than other technologies and partial bonding of the filament layers and voids in the mesostructures due to the tubular filament nature

finish that precludes reasonable resistance to catheter insertions, models require infiltration with an appropriate sealant to become watertight, which can alter the intended anatomy.

Material extrusion is nonetheless favored by early 3D printing labs because it is overall economical and easy to use; materials tend to be more rugged and strong than previously described technologies and cost less than $100/kg. Large build platforms with maximum dimensions of roughly 91 × 61 × 91 cm are readily commercially available at smaller cost than comparable size printers for other technologies. In general, this technology is not optimal for anatomic modeling applications such as surgical planning and simulation, except for musculoskeletal printing for orthopedic applications, since large bones can be printed at lower cost and reduced post-processing than with other technologies. However, assistive technology providers may prefer this technology due to the higher strength of the materials. In the future, we expect it to be most useful for the printing of patient-specific guides and surgical tools due to material strength, biocompatibility, and cost. Finally, many advances in this technology are currently underway to create parts with more isotropic characteristics.

2.1.2.5 Powder Bed Fusion

This category of 3D printing technologies includes selective laser sintering (SLS), direct metal laser sintering (DMLS), selective laser melting (SLM), and electron beam melting (EBM). These technologies generally use a high-power laser or electron beam to fuse small particles of plastic, metal, ceramic, or glass that is held in a tray in powder form. The powder is typically pre-heated to just below the material melting point. The target of the energy source is then controlled by the printer, allowing it to selectively fuse or melt the powder at each successive layer on the surface of the powder bed. After a layer is fused, the powder bed is lowered by one layer thickness, and a new powder layer is laid on top by a roller, and the next layer is printed. Like binder jetting, most of the nonmetal materials in powder bed fusion technologies do not require support structures since the model is always fully surrounded and supported by unsintered powder. However, metal materials may require supports to transfer heat away from the part and reduce swelling during the printing process. The support bed enables powder bed fusion printers to construct 3D geometries such as a lattice, useful for implants that promote osseointegration not readily possible with other methods.

Powder bed fusion technologies are used extensively for 3D printing of medical devices including implants, fixations, and surgical tools and guides (Fig. 2.11). Specifically, material groups compatible with the technology are

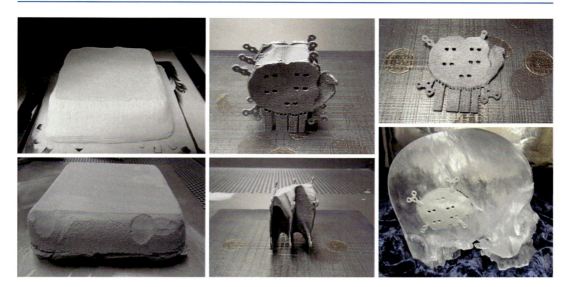

Fig. 2.11 Model 3D printed using a metal powder bed fusion printer. After printing the model is encased in the powder (*left-hand column*). After removal from powder (*middle column*), the cranial plate is cleaned and placed on a model of the patient's skull to confirm fit (*right-hand column*)

synthetic polymers (e.g., nylon, polyether ether ketone [PEKK]) and metals (e.g., titanium and cobalt-chrome alloys) that are biocompatible and sterilizable and can be safely implanted. Bioresorbable materials that can be printed with these printers offer exciting advances for patient-specific temporary devices such as splints (Morrison et al. 2015). The print material that is used may dictate the usefulness for anatomic models. For example, for a model used for presurgical planning, metal would most likely not be a useful (or acceptable) material. Metal parts would primarily be used for implants, guides, and surgical tools. Nylon models are versatile and possess good mechanical properties and heat resistance that allows for parts to be drilled or sawed with surgical instruments without melting. However, accuracy of most powder bed fusion machines is less than that of vat photopolymerization and material jetting machines.

Powder bed fusion materials are expensive, exceeding $200/kg, and some metals can exceed $400/kg. The rate-limiting steps of this technology are largely dictated by machine thermal cycles and model post-processing (Fig. 2.11). Many of these machines need to heat to a desired temperature to print, and parts need to cool before the operator can remove them from the machine. Required post-processing steps are highly dependent on the particular technique/material. For example, heat hardening/residual stress relaxation may be required for metals. Metal parts may need to be released/cut from the build platform, and finished parts may require computer numerical control (CNC) milling to achieve smooth, polished surfaces. One of the most significant hurdles when using this technology for medical devices is the difficulty of ensuring that unsintered powder remaining in printed model cavities will not affect biocompatibility and sterilization, especially in lattice-type structures (Di Prima et al. 2016).

2.1.2.6 Other Technologies

Three additional technologies are discussed in this section that are not currently encountered in medical 3D printing applications. The first is a newly developed technique introduced by Hewlett Packard, termed Multi Jet Fusion. This technology shares elements of both powder bed fusion and binder jetting technologies. It jets both a fusing and a detailing (inhibiting) agent on a bed of powder, which are activated with energy (heat) to fuse (rather than bind) the raw powder material. This technique promises multicolor printing, exceptional part strength, and the ability to introduce texture internally within printed parts. It appears this technology has applications for medical modeling, but printers are only at pre-commercial release as of this writing.

The other two technologies, sheet lamination and directed energy deposition, have limited medical applications. Sheet lamination is an inexpensive 3D printing method that bonds paper, metal, or plastic film. Each sheet is rolled/pulled onto the build tray, and then a knife or laser cutter traces the outline of the shape of the printed object at the layer of the object being printed; glue and/or a heat treatment is applied between the layers for adherence to the previous layer. The sheet can be pre-printed with color to produce colored models. Post-processing involves the removal of excess material, by manually peeling off geometry not included in the printed model. This may not be easy (or possible) for complex anatomic geometries, such as cavities or areas surrounding tortuous structures such as vessels. Paper sheet lamination may however be economical for some orthopedic applications where only the outer bone surface needs to be evaluated. Additional post-processing by infiltration with a sealant or wax may be appropriate for paper models. Although this technology is generally cheaper than other processes, the printing and post-processing time may be extensive. Finally, directed energy deposition directly deposits material to a location where a high-powered energy source is also directed to melt/fuse the material. This technology combines aspects of material extrusion and powder bed fusion (laser or electron beam) and offers metal printing. It is unique because it can add to or repair an existing part, but this option is likely of limited use in medical applications.

2.1.3 3D Printer Resolution, Accuracy, and Reproducibility

In general, the highest resolution achievable by 3D printing modalities in all three axes is roughly 0.05–0.1 mm, superior to the resolution of images created by most clinical imaging modalities. For 3D printers, the z-axis resolution (layer thickness) is typically considered separately from the x–y plane resolution and is the most commonly encountered "resolution" figure found in literature. Similar to slice thickness in medical imaging systems, layer thickness is user selectable for most printers, and, similar to medical imaging protocols where slice thickness directly affects scan time, its choice directly affects printing time. If thinner layers are chosen, the print heads or energy sources will need to trace proportionally more layers, and the print will require a proportionally longer time. Partly because of its effect on printing time, layer thickness is the dimension of lowest resolution of 3D printers.

Of note however is that currently most printer's layer thickness is less than that of most medical CT images. Material extrusion printers print at typically 0.1–0.4 mm layer thickness; vat photopolymerization printers have 0.02–0.2 mm layer thickness; material jetting can print layers as small as 16 μm thick; and binder jetting layer thicknesses are typically 0.05–0.1 mm. Unlike imaging systems, where slice thickness can usually be arbitrarily large, for 3D printers, the layer thickness has an upper limit, and this upper limit may be dependent on the material being used to print. For example, a laser cannot penetrate a resin that uses a pigment for color to the same extent as it can a clear resin, and in either case penetration depth is limited. Although laser power is automatically adjusted by an SLA printer based on the resin being used, there are limits which, for example, might allow a 0.2 mm maximum layer thickness for a clear resin and a 0.1 mm maximum thickness for a colored resin. Similar implications exist for other technologies, for example, infiltration of a powder by the jetted binder in a binder jet system.

Most 3D printers have a fixed resolution in the x–y axes that is not as immediately clear in literature and requires some interpretation of equipment specifications. In SLA and SLS printers, x–y resolution is determined by the laser beam spot size (diameter), which is roughly 0.1–0.2 mm for most commercial systems. For DLP printers, it is determined by the projector resolution, optics, and build platform size. One measure used to convey resolution of DLP printers is the number of dots per inch (dpi). The higher the dpi, the better the x–y plane resolution of the printer. A printer with 800 dpi has 800 individually controlled dots of the printing source (e.g., individual print head or energy source target points) with which to print 1 in. (25.4 mm) of the model. This printer thus has an in-plane "resolution" of 0.03175 mm. DPI is also commonly used to measure binder jet and material jetting printer resolutions, which typically lie in the 600–1200 dpi range.

Importantly, despite the high resolution of printers mentioned above, models usually cannot be printed successfully with features <0.3 mm in size (George et al 2017a). The minimum size of a feature that can be successfully printed depends on the printing technology and is often only partly dependent on the printer's in-plane resolution. For example, the minimum feature size is roughly 1.5 times the laser beam spot size (x–y resolution) for SLA printers. For material and binder jet printers, jetted droplets have distinct dimensional tolerances and spread characteristics that affect minimum feature size beyond the stated printer dpi. For these two technologies, manufacturers typically indicate the minimum feature size, which is usually 0.1–0.3 mm.

Resolution is the smallest scale that a 3D printer can reproduce and is only one factor affecting accuracy. Certainly, models can only be as accurate as the lowest resolution of the printer in each of the three axes (typically the z-axis layer thickness); a model printed with a printer operating at 0.4 mm layer thickness cannot be accurate to less than 0.4 mm compared to the intended medical model. In contrast to resolution, accuracy refers to the degree of agreement between the dimensions of the printed object compared to those intended, i.e., the dimensions of the digital object as stored in the STL file (Liacouras 2017). The accuracy and reproducibility of 3D printing medical models has unfortunately not been thoroughly investigated to date. Chapter 11 further discusses accuracy, reproducibility, and quality of medical 3D printing.

2.2 3D Printing Materials

Most printer manufacturers, and for many printers, third parties offer a choice of materials for use with each machine. Different materials are formulated for different needs, for example, low-cost prototyping, strength for tools, color, and biocompatibility. Many printing materials have undergone testing for US Pharmacopeial Convention (USP) Class VI or International Standards Organization (ISO) 10993, referring to levels of minimal in vivo biological reactivity (FDA 2016). These materials may be generally preferred, but are likely not necessary for models for surgical planning, teaching, and patient-physician interaction purposes. The use of materials that meet the requirements of those standards is however required to produce surgical guides and tools. Metals such as titanium and cobalt-chrome alloys can be used to print implants and implantable devices, and nylon can be used to print surgical guides. These are primarily printed with powder bed fusion and rarely material extrusion technologies.

Many printing materials can be sterilized for intraoperative use. Appropriate sterilization techniques depend on the material and may involve steam, chemical, and radiation sterilization (Mitsouras et al. 2015). At present, 3D printer and material manufacturers generally provide sterilization recommendations for appropriate materials. Generally, printed guides and implants will require ethylene oxide or other non-heat sterilization such as gamma radiation, while metal and some nylons can withstand autoclaving.

2.3 Conclusions

To date, medical researchers and clinicians have had limited access to and knowledge of the underlying 3D printing technologies. This is rapidly changing, and many surgery and radiology practices are starting their own 3D printing labs. Knowledge of the capabilities and limitations of the various 3D printing technologies is key to successful investment and foray into medical 3D printing.

As demonstrated in this chapter, each printer technology may have its own optimal application(s); therefore, before a facility decides to invest large capital to purchase a 3D printer, it would be beneficial for them to decide what their focus will be. Three-dimensional printers to date require manual intervention from an experienced user to properly manufacture parts and maintain the machines. Additional considerations include the diagnostic imaging processing software to produce STL models, and computer-assisted design software that allows 3D digital model processing and optimization for printing, or to plan surgical reconstruction. These are also large investments and require additional trained operators.

The potential medical uses of three-dimensional printing may only be limited by one's imagination. Imagination, however, is only one aspect of a successful implementation. Interdisciplinary communication and collaboration, knowledge exchange, and a firm grasp of the technological advances are essential to the successful implementation of medical 3D printing toward enhancing the expert care provided to patients.

References

Chepelev L, Giannopoulos AA, Tang A, Mitsouras D, Rybicki FJ. Medical 3D printing: methods to standardize terminology and report trends. 3D Print Med. 2017;3:4.

Di Prima M, Coburn J, Hwang D, Kelly J, Khairuzzaman A, Ricles L. Additively manufactured medical products – the FDA perspective. 3D Print Med. 2016;2:1.

Fishman EK, Drebin B, Magid D, et al. Volumetric rendering techniques: applications for three-dimensional imaging of the hip. Radiology. 1987;163(3):737–8.

George E, Liacouras, G. E, Rybicki FJ, Mitsouras D. Measuring and establishing the accuracy & reproducibility of 3D-printed medical models. Radiographics. 2017a; doi:10.1148/rg.2017160165.

George E, Liacouras P, Lee TC, Mitsouras D. 3D-printed patient-specific models for CT- and MRI-guided procedure planning. Am J Neuroradiol. 2017b; doi:10.3174/ajnr.A5189.

Giannopoulos AA, Steigner ML, George E, et al. Cardiothoracic applications of 3-dimensional printing. J Thorac Imaging. 2016;31(5):253–72.

Guenette JP, Himes N, Giannopoulos AA, Kelil T, Mitsouras D, Lee TC. Computer-based vertebral tumor cryoablation planning and procedure simulation involving two cases using MRI-visible 3D printing and advanced visualization. Am J Roentgenol. 2016;207(5):1128–31.

Hiller J, Lipson H. STL 2.0: a proposal for a universal multi-material Additive Manufacturing File format. Proc Solid Freeform Fabrication Symposium (SFF'09), Austin, Texas 2009; p. 266–78.

Huang Y, Leu MC. NSF Additive Manufacturing Workshop Report. NSF workshop on frontiers of additive manufacturing research and education. Arlington, VA: University of Florida Center for Manufacturing Innovation; 2013.

ISO 17296-2:2015. Additive manufacturing – general principles – Part 2: Overview of process categories and feedstock. Geneva: International Organization for Standardization; 2015.

ISO/ASTM52915 - 16. Standard specification for additive manufacturing file format (AMF) version 1.2. Book of standards. West Conshohocken, PA: ASTM International; 2016.

Mayer R, Liacouras P, Thomas A, Kang M, Lin L, Simone CB II. 3D printer generated thorax phantom with mobile tumor for radiation dosimetry. Rev Sci Instrum. 2015;86(7):074301.

Mitsouras D, Liacouras P, Imanzadeh A, et al. Medical 3D printing for the radiologist. Radiographics. 2015;35(7):1965–88.

Mitsouras D, Lee TC, Liacouras P, et al. Three-dimensional printing of MRI-visible phantoms and MR image-guided therapy simulation. Magn Reson Med. 2017;77(2):613–22.

Morrison RJ, Hollister SJ, Niedner MF, et al. Mitigation of tracheobronchomalacia with 3D-printed personalized medical devices in pediatric patients. Sci Transl Med. 2015;7(285):285ra64.

Rubin GD, Dake MD, Napel SA, McDonnell CH, Jeffrey RB Jr. Three-dimensional spiral CT angiography of the abdomen: initial clinical experience. Radiology. 1993;186(1):147–52.

Tumbleston JR, Shirvanyants D, Ermoshkin N, et al. Additive manufacturing. Continuous liquid interface production of 3D objects. Science. 2015;347(6228):1349–52.

U.S. Department of Health and Human Services—Food and Drug Administration Center for Devices and Radiological Health. Use of International Standard ISO 10993-1, "Biological evaluation of medical devices - Part 1: Evaluation and testing within a risk management process". Washington DC: U.S. Department of Health and Human Services; 2016.

Post-processing of DICOM Images

3

Andreas A. Giannopoulos and Todd Pietila

3.1 Introduction

Medical three-dimensional (3D) printing of human anatomy and pathology begins with the acquisition of 3D volumetric imaging data wherein the tissues of interest have sufficient contrast/signal intensity to be differentiated (Mitsouras et al. 2015). The process of fabricating a 3D-printed physical model involves a number of steps that can be best described as a medley of medical imaging, image post-processing, and industrial-level manufacturing. Post-processing of Digital Imaging and Communications in Medicine (DICOM) imaging data is an essential and necessary step to enable the manufacturing of both patient-specific 3D-printed models and medical devices. The requirements of this workflow differ from traditional image post-processing techniques as it requires the generation of a suitable digital file format that is compatible with 3D printers.

A.A. Giannopoulos, M.D. (✉)
Cardiac Imaging, Department of Nuclear Medicine,
University Hospital Zurich,
Raemistrasse 100, 8091 Zurich, Switzerland

Applied Imaging Science Lab, Radiology
Department, Brigham and Women's Hospital,
Harvard Medical School, 75 Francis Street, MA
02115 Boston, USA
e-mail: andgiannop@hotmail.com

T. Pietila, B.Sc.
Materialise USA, 44650 Helm Court,
Plymouth, MI 48170, USA

The actual 3D printing process refers to the fabrication of a tangible object from this digital file by a 3D printer. Materials are commonly deposited layer by layer and then fused to form the final 3D object. Additive manufacturing (AM), rapid prototyping (RP), and additive fabrication (AF) are synonyms for 3D printing. According to the most recent classification by American Society of Testing and Materials (ASTM), there are seven major types of 3D printing technology (ASTM 2014; Huang and Leu 2013). Although these technologies share similarities, they differ in speed, cost, and resolution of the product as detailed in Chap. 2.

A handheld 3D-printed model derived from DICOM images represents a natural progression from 3D visualization. DICOM image files cannot be used directly for 3D printing; further steps are necessary to make them readable by 3D printers. In summary, these steps include image segmentation, Standard Tessellation Language (STL) file generation, and computer-aided design (CAD) modeling for refinement or instrument/device design, model quality check, and file fixing (Fig. 3.1).

Decisions made in each stage of the process will be driven by several factors including the imaging modality used, the anatomy modeled, and the intended use of the eventual 3D-printed model. Some of the initial post-processing steps may be familiar to the medical imaging experts, as they share common features with 3D visualization tools that are used for image post-

F.J. Rybicki, G.T. Grant (eds.), *3D Printing in Medicine*, DOI 10.1007/978-3-319-61924-8_3

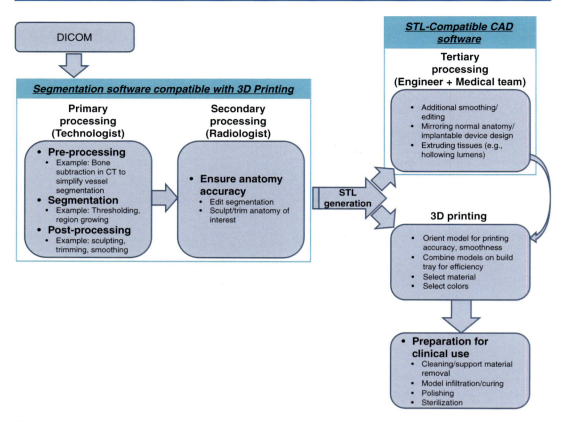

Fig. 3.1 Flowchart shows sample workflow for a radiology-centered 3D three-dimensional printing process. Digital Imaging and Communications in Medicine (DICOM) images are initially processed with compatible segmentation software, and the segmented anatomy is reviewed by the radiologist. An STL file of the selected tissues is then generated. The anatomic parts defined in the STL file can be 3D printed or further manipulated with compatible CAD computer-aided design software to, for example, design prostheses or produce a support platform to hold the parts in place. Final preparation of the tangible 3D-printed model (e.g., cleaning and sterilization) is required before clinical use. Reprinted with permission from Mitsouras et al., Radiographics. 2015

processing tasks. However, bridging the imaging data to 3D printing technologies requires an extra set of steps for refining and proper manipulation of the 3D rendering and finally preparing it for 3D printing.

Typically, manipulating DICOM images for 3D printing involves accurate segmentation of the desired tissues via placement of regions of interest (ROIs), followed by creation and refinement of the STL representation of the ensemble surfaces defined by those ROIs. The refinement step is new to imagers and generally requires specialized software and skills used primarily in engineering applications. The operator must also carefully review the final STL model against source images for ensuring quality and accuracy.

A number of free and commercial software are available to achieve these steps, namely, image segmentation with STL file generation and CAD-based STL manipulations. Examples are Vitrea (Vital Images, Inc., Minnetonka, MN) and OsiriX (Pixmeo, Geneva, Switzerland) for the former task and Geomagic Freeform (3D Systems, Rock Hill, NC) or Meshmixer (Autodesk, Inc., San Rafael, CA) for STL manipulations. Although these are two distinct categories of software, medical 3D printing software suites exist such as the Mimics Innovation Suite (Materialise, Leuven, Belgium) and Mimics inPrint (Materialise, Leuven, Belgium) that provide a solution combining elements of DICOM image processing and digital CAD.

3.2   Image Segmentation

Imaging modalities utilized for medical 3D printing commonly involve high-resolution, cross-sectional imaging, most commonly computed tomography (CT) (Mitsouras et al. 2015; Greil et al. 2007; Schmauss et al. 2015) and magnetic resonance imaging (MRI) (Greil et al. 2007; Yoo et al. 2016). More recently, success has been reported with the use of ultrasound in the cardiovascular field with the use of 3D transthoracic echocardiography (TTE) and transesophageal echocardiography (TEE) (Mahmood et al. 2015; Olivieri et al. 2015). Finally, rotational digital subtraction angiography or 3D rotational angiography has also been employed (Frolich et al. 2016; Ionita et al. 2011; Poterucha et al. 2014). It has also been demonstrated that multiple imaging modalities can be used to create a hybrid 3D-printed model enabled by the imaging strengths of each modality. For example, combining CT with TEE has been employed for generation of a 3D model of the heart capturing both structural and valve morphology (Gosnell et al. 2016).

Sufficient "pre-print" planning taking into account the modality and the parameters to be selected for source image data acquisition increases the accuracy and ease of the printed model; the quality of the images is tethered with the quality of the model. Optimizing spatial and temporal resolution along with appropriate contrast in structures of interest will result in the highest-quality models and most efficient data processing (Fig. 3.2).

Generally, the thinner the image cross sections (e.g., commonly reported 0.5–1.25 mm for cardiac 3D printing) (Jacobs et al. 2008), the more accurate the delineation of anatomical structures given the enhanced spatial resolution, yet very thin slices can lead to cumbersome post-processing and are not always recommended. Importantly, the desired image quality should be identified by selecting appropriate image reconstruction techniques, such as reconstruction kernels; smooth kernels generate images with lower noise but with reduced spatial resolution, while sharp kernels generate images with higher spatial resolution, bounded though with increased noise (Flohr et al. 2007; Matsumoto et al. 2015). After acquiring imaging in the appropriate resolution and quality, segmentation of these DICOM images is the first step toward manufacturing a patient-specific 3D-printed model.

A number of software programs and algorithms are available to perform image segmentation which can often be tailored toward specific imaging protocols or anatomy. The segmentation of appropriate ROIs can be both automated and

CT
Poor spatial resolution

MRI
Poor contrast

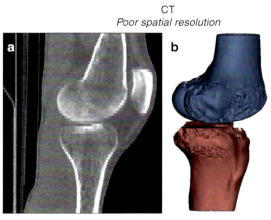
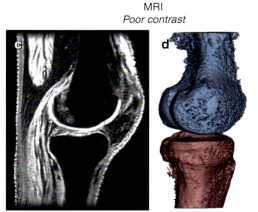

Fig. 3.2 Examples of poor raw image data quality for generating 3D printable files. Panels (**a**) and (**b**) show a reconstructed STL file of the femur and tibia from a CT scan with 3 mm slice increment resulting in low resolution and missing data in the reconstruction. Panels (**c**) and (**d**) demonstrate STL files of femur and tibia derived from a T2-weighted MRI with poor contrast between the bone and surrounding soft tissue

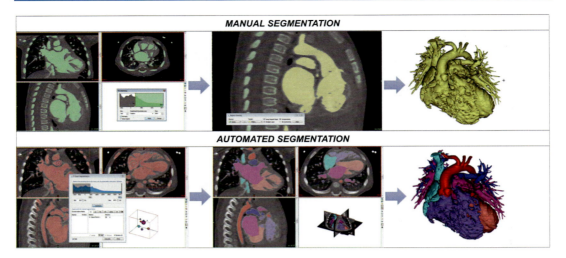

Fig. 3.3 Paradigms of manual vs. automated segmentation in a case of double outlet right ventricle. *Upper panels* show the process of manual segmentation that involve thresholding, region growing, and generation of a single STL file including the entirety of the heart and the great vessels. *Lower panels* demonstrate the automated approach to segment the same case using automated algorithms for thresholding, separating the heart chambers and the great vessels and providing a composite STL model

manual or more frequently semiautomated, combining an initial step of automated segmentation followed by manual corrections (Fig. 3.3).

Automated algorithms include thresholding, edge detection, and region growing. In thresholding, a widely used technique, voxels in the tissue of interest are selected based on the range of intensity values of that tissue (Mitsouras et al. 2015). Although this technique suffices for bone segmentation from CT because the HU are higher than surrounding structures, more complex algorithms are usually necessary, such as dynamic adjustment of the thresholding range. This is especially the case when processing MRI data where the pixel gray values do not correlate with tissue density. Common imaging artifacts also require interpretation and manual corrections. For example, due to noise or beam hardening in a CT image, a portion of an enhanced vessel lumen may fall outside of the typical enhanced blood HU range. If dynamic region growing or hole filling is not performed, the printed model may contain a nonanatomical hole or void. A segmentation approach such as "wrapping" of a segmented region can also be used in such cases or to fill true anatomic voids such as in the cancellous bone to produce a simple solid model (Harrysson et al. 2007; Kozakiewicz et al.

2009). Additionally, metal artifact from implants or dental fillings causes streaking artifact which is challenging to handle with automated segmentation processes (Fig. 3.4).

Region selection (also called region growing) is a useful second step to determine whether segmented voxels belong to "a single or multiple" parts to be 3D printed. Region growing typically reduces the burden of the final step, namely, manual editing ("sculpting") of the 3D ROIs that surround the segmented voxels, which includes manually manipulating ROI boundaries and manually erasing, combining, and modifying parts.

It is important to recognize that a 3D-printed model cannot convey information regarding tissues that are either not visualized in the imaging modality used to acquire the source images or that do not have sufficient differences in signal or density from adjacent tissues. For example, nerves are not clearly delineated on a standard CT; thus, it would be challenging to create a 3D model demonstrating the relationship of the brachial plexus to a superior sulcus tumor. This can be overcome by placing geometric objects (i.e., splines) to represent the paths of nerves or small vessels when they are not easily segmented from the source images. It is also possible to fuse imaging data from

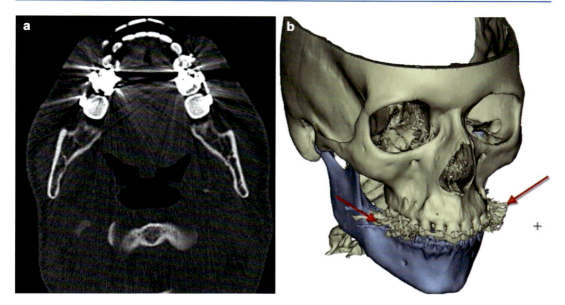

Fig. 3.4 (**a**, **b**) Streaking artifact in CT imaging resulting from metal in the body. Manual segmentation processing is typically required to counter the artifact and generate an accurate 3D reconstruction

multiple imaging modalities to create such a model, for example, the bone and vasculature can be visualized in a contrast-enhanced CT and the nerves in an MRI of the brachial plexus.

One typically segments only those tissues visualized in the images that are relevant to convey to clinicians. For example, in a case of chest wall tumor, the adjacent portion of the rib cage and the vascular supply may be deemed pertinent to print in addition to the tumor itself, but not the mediastinal structures which are outside the surgical field or the non-adherent lung which does not pose a surgical challenge. This is necessary not only because segmentation is a time-consuming and currently laborious task but also because the efficacy and thus clinical utility of the model hinge on its ability to quickly communicate the relevant information. Thus, while an anterior mediastinal mass model could contain the entire rib cage and thoracic spine, the resulting model would likely present difficulties in clear visualization of the tumor and for comprehension of the relationship of the tumor to more crucial mediastinal structures. In this context, 3D printing of complex models at present also demands an artistic component, since no guidelines have been clearly established as to what

tissues are useful to include in a model for any one particular indication (Giannopoulos et al. 2016). Future work should aim to optimize this aspect of this new modality.

3.3   STL Generation

Since tissues are segmented by demarcating their boundaries in individual, successive 2D cross-sectional images that compose a 3D image volume, the next step required is to assemble a 3D representation of the tissue and produce a closed surface "shell" of each tissue from its individually demarcated 2D cross sections. This shell is almost universally a surface mesh composed of small triangles and stored as a STL file format. The STL file format is to 3D printers what the DICOM format is to radiology workstations. Workstation software knows how to interpret the signal values stored in DICOM files so as to display them as an image on a monitor. Similarly, 3D printer drivers know how to interpret the triangles in an STL file so as to manufacture the physical object enclosed by them.

Figure 3.5 illustrates the process of generating an STL model.

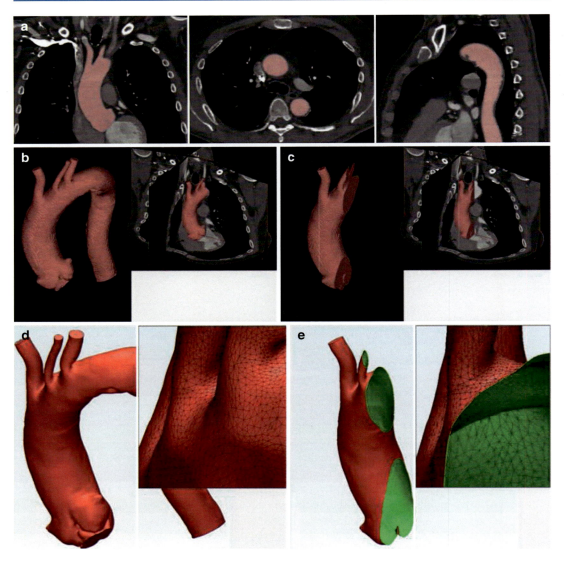

Fig. 3.5 Generation of a 3D-printable STL model from a volumetric medical image dataset. The aorta and aortic arch vessels are first segmented from a contrast-enhanced CT (**a**). The segmented image voxels identify the region of space occupied by blood, and conversely this region of space is entirely filled by the individually segmented voxels (**b**). If one were to cut through this region, it would simply expose the inner voxels that have been segmented (**c**). An STL model that can be 3D printed is instead a surface composed of small triangles that enclose the segmented voxels (**d**; shown in *red*, with individual triangle outlines shown in *inset*). Cutting this surface merely exposes the inner side of the triangles (**e**; shown in *green*, with individual triangle outlines shown in *inset*). Reprinted with permission from Giannopoulos et al., J Thor Imag. 2016

Once segmentation of the DICOM images has been performed, the voxel data must be converted to a 3D surface file recognizable by digital CAD software and 3D printers. Many of the image segmentation software will have the ability to convert the segmented images to a tessellated surface file most commonly using an implementation of the marching cubes algorithm. After segmentation, most software packages generate a printable 3D STL model of the surfaces surrounding segmented tissues based on algorithms such as interpolation and pattern recognition that preserve anatomical

Fig. 3.6 STL of a femur generated from a volumetric medical image dataset. The *top* femur is reconstructed with more triangles thus preserving more detail. The *bottom* femur reconstructed with fewer triangle thus resulting in a disfeatured, less accurate 3D model

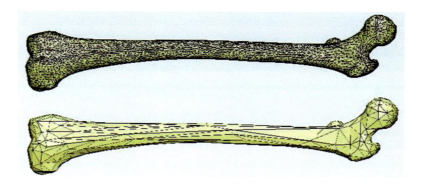

Table 3.1 Recommended number of triangles for 3D printing different anatomical models

Anatomical model	Maximum triangles[a]
Skull	600,000
Face	450,000
Mandible	200,000
Femur	300,000
Full spine	850,000

Reprinted with permission from Mitsouras et al., Radiographics. 2015
[a]Note finer detail models (i.e., vascular) may require a higher triangle count

features. The easiest way to understand this step is as follows: using ROIs, operators select voxels that enclose a 3D surface. Conversion of this surface to STL can use any number of triangular facets to fit these surfaces; too few will compromise anatomical features in the 3D-printed model, while too many leads to unnecessary roughness in the object if the segmented surface is not smooth (Fig. 3.6). In our experience, STL-based models have no benefit to the provider once they exceed a given threshold of triangles for some common models (Mitsouras et al. 2015) (Table 3.1).

3.4   Computer-Aided Design Software

Although most 3D visualization software packages have the ability to save the segmentation, process the segmented surfaces, and export them as an STL file, for the majority of medical applications, this STL conversion is suboptimal due to segmentation imperfections. A simple example is a coronary artery CT angiogram segmented as consecutive cross-sectional ROIs. The collection of ROIs defines a surface that can be volume rendered. However, it cannot be printed because it is "open." By this we mean that where the segmented vessel ends or is in any way incomplete (e.g., the branch vessels), to a 3D printer this ROI surface has no physical meaning and cannot be printed because it does not enclose a volume of space. This "closing" is one example of the "STL refinement" step that produces the final product sent for 3D printing.

Other manipulations include fixing errors such as holes (e.g., gaps between triangular facets), inverted normals (defining what is inside versus outside the part to be printed), and applying local and/or global smoothing of the model. In this step, the design of additional parts is performed, for example, the design of implants, or adding supports to hold parts of the printed model in place. Such alterations are unique to preparing anatomical models for 3D printing and separate it from 3D visualization.

3.5   Model Refinement and CAD Design

CAD software specifically designed to handle mesh-based geometries is required as traditional parametric CAD software will not handle complex anatomical surface models. The necessary CAD functions and workflow will differ depending on the case and the intended use of the model. This can include adding fixtures to incorporate the model into a testing or simulation environment, cutting anatomy to achieve internal visualization of organs, virtual planning, and custom instrument or device design.

The refinements to the 3D surface file often require operations such as cutting, smoothing, adding connector supports, and designing features to hold the anatomy in a desired position or integrate with an existing test apparatus (Fig. 3.7) (Friedman et al. 2016).

For modeling complex congenital heart cases, for example, it is often desired by the surgeon to visualize the complexities of the intracardiac anatomy (Giannopoulos et al. 2015). In order to achieve this visualization, the heart must be virtually cut in order to open these desired windows in the anatomy. For building multi-organ system models, often spaces will be left between neighboring organs. In order to hold these organs in the proper position after printing, connecting supports can be added with CAD software. Another application of using CAD software to manipulate an anatomical model is preparing a model to integrate with an existing test or simulation fixture. For example, performing endovascular

interventional procedures in a simulation environment has shown the ability to predict the proper devices and techniques for a patient. These models are often plugged into a pump system or positioned under fluoroscopy in the catheterization lab environment. In order to plug the model into a fluid pump or position properly on a table, inlet/outlet connectors need to be added in addition to a baseplate to properly register the anatomy.

3.6 Virtual Procedural Planning

Virtual procedural planning has also become commonplace and the gold standard for specialties in dentistry, craniomaxillofacial, and orthopedic surgery. Surgical planning using 3D reconstructed models has inherent benefits in that it leverages three dimensions resulting in a more precise surgical plan. Dedicated software tools exist for planning and simulating surgical outcomes by manipulating the reconstructed anatomical geometries. This allows a clinician to

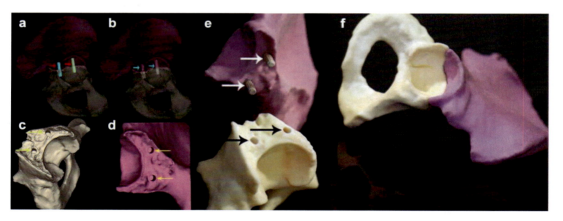

Fig. 3.7 CAD manipulation of models using a case of a transverse acetabular fracture with upper and lower fragments. Panels (**a**)–(**d**) demonstrate the CAD modeling, whereas panels (**e**) and (**f**) show the actual 3D-printed model. (**a**) The colored pegs (*red arrows*) are sized 0.5 mm larger than fluted dowels and placed in a parallel orientation across both superior and inferior parts of the fracture. They are then subtracted out of both "shells" of the fracture using a Boolean operation (notice holes in part (**b**), *blue arrows*). (**c, d**) This results in hollow cylinders that could be printed in the final part (*yellow arrows*), which allows the parts be connected with fluted dowels, for a "press fit," allowing the user to separate and connect the object multiple times, much like a puzzle piece, and inspect each piece individually as well as a whole. (**e**) Demonstrates the holes which were created virtually and into the part (*black arrow*). Fluted dowels fit tightly into the holes (*white arrow*) and allow the two pieces to remain together without being held (as seen in **f**), but also come apart. Reprinted with permission from Friedman et al., Skeletal Radiol 2016

Fig. 3.8 Virtual surgery. Demonstrates a virtual correction of malunion of a radius. (**a**) Note the angles measured along the 3D surface of the deformity. Virtual cutting objects are made at the appropriate angles (**b**), and then the radius malunion is virtually corrected (**c**), and the final proposed plan is shown (**d**). This can aid surgeons in deciding how to perform the osteotomy. Cutting jigs can be made for the surgeon to use intraoperatively, obviating the osteotomies freehand. Reprinted with permission from Friedman et al., Skeletal Radiol 2016

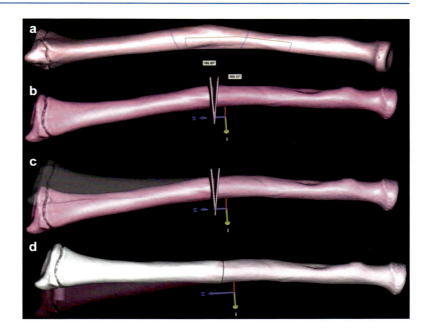

perform virtual osteotomies and repositioning of bone or determine optimal locations for plating (Fig. 3.8). These are often performed in collaboration with a clinical engineer and result in the design and manufacturing of custom cutting and drilling guides to execute the planned procedure.

The impact of medical 3D printing is often the highest when it can be leveraged to design and manufacture a custom implant to treat a patient not suitable for an off-the-shelf implant. CAD design software is essential in this step to design a device-specific fitting to a patient's reconstructed anatomy. This has been demonstrated in the creation of custom cranial prosthesis, orthopedic joint replacement, and even implantable tracheal splints.

3.7 Model Quality

When 3D models have an intended use of planning or executing a procedure, additional quality measures should take place during the software modeling workflow. As a result of the multistage process, errors can be created and propagated as a dataset is processed. This can include oversmoothing of anatomy (Fig. 3.9), removal of

pertinent structures, and scaling errors between software.

As a practice, it is important to verify the accuracy of the processed surface file prior to 3D printing. This can be done subjectively by overlaying the 3D surface model back on top of the DICOM image slices enabling a visual verification of the model accuracy in the relevant areas. Additionally, traceability can be important for a center producing high volumes of 3D-printed models with often multiple models being printed on a single build. By stamping the 3D model with a unique identifier, it will ensure that the model is delivered to the proper clinician and patient case.

3.8 Preparation for 3D Printing

Reconstructed surface files are not created equal in quality or printability. In order to successfully build a model on a 3D printer, it must be free of errors and considered "watertight" or free of holes in the mesh surface. This requires a verification and fixing step to ensure the quality is appropriate and the file is prepared for printing. Removal of noise shells, intersect-

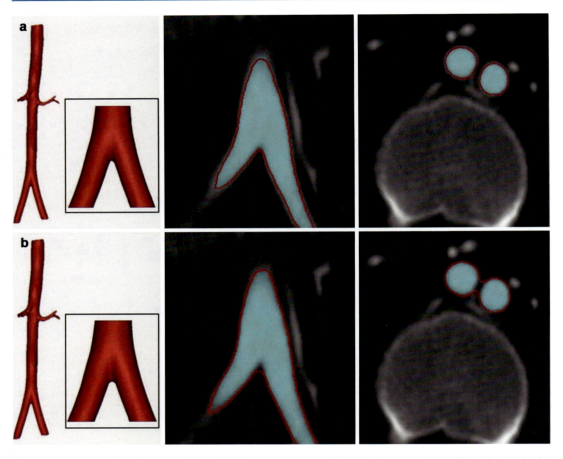

Fig. 3.9 Post-processing of contrast-enhanced CT images of the abdominal aorta. (**a**) On coronal (*middle*) and axial (*right*) CT images, the aorta is segmented by using thresholding (*turquoise* in **a** and **b**), and an enclosing STL surface (3D rendition on *left* and *red outlines* in **a** and **b**) is generated. (**b**) On the coronal (*middle*) and axial (*right*) CT images, subsequent refinement of the STL file by using standard smoothing and wrapping operations may no longer correctly describe the anatomy. Reprinted with permission from Mitsouras et al., Radiographics. 2015

ing elements, and holes are all important to ensure a successful build. Depending on the 3D printing technology chosen, it may also be useful to perform wall thickness verification and repair to the geometry. If structures in the model are smaller than the resolution of the 3D printer, it will result in missing or poorly represented structures. In addition, many 3D-printed materials become brittle or tear sensitive at smaller dimensions. Software is available to analyze and repair the part with these considerations in mind. Lastly, build orientation and printer setup need to be performed. This is a unique process with each 3D printing technology and vendor.

3.9 Special Applications

Alternate data capturing modalities are also suitable for applications of medical 3D printing which include 3D imaging systems that are uncommon in medical facilities. These systems include laser, optical, and photogrammetry 3D scanning systems which capture surface geometry from an object and enable a digital representation to be created by projecting a light source or laser to collect the data points representing the surface morphology. Surface scanning is popular for 3D printing applications where enhanced resolution is required or for modeling that require only skin surface data. One example is for planning orthognathic surgery where a high-resolution optical scan of the patient's teeth can help plan the optimal correction and teeth occlusion. Additionally, prosthetists use surface scanning equipment to create custom facial and other external prosthetic devices.

3.10 Conclusions

3D printing is considered to hold key role in medical imaging in the years to come and is expected to improve medical care. Post-processing of DICOM images represents the cornerstone of transforming two-dimensional cross-sectional images to three-dimensional physical models. Accuracy and reproducibility of the 3D printing models depend on multiple factors including operator's segmentation expertise and ability to interpret human anatomy and pathology in the source images, all the more in different modalities. These technical aspects are important to address and work is currently underway (Cai et al. 2015; Olivieri et al. 2015). Existing image segmentation methods remain rather laborious, and more efforts should be made toward automatization of the process (Byrne et al. 2016; Tandon et al. 2016). As medical imaging, software tools, and 3D printing equipment improve in speed and quality along with a greater selection of materials, new opportunities will present.

References

(ASTM), A. S. F. T. A. M. F2792-12a Standard terminology for additive manufacturing technologies. In: Electronics; declarable substances in materials; 3D imaging systems. West Conshohocken, PA: ASTM; 2014.

Byrne N, Velasco Forte M, Tandon A, Valverde I, Hussain T. A systematic review of image segmentation methodology, used in the additive manufacture of patient-specific 3D printed models of the cardiovascular system. JRSM Cardiovasc Dis. 2016;5:2048004016645467.

Cai T, Rybicki F, Giannopoulos A, Schultz K, Kumamaru K, Liacouras P, Demehri S, Shu Small K, Mitsouras D. The residual STL volume as a metric to evaluate accuracy and reproducibility of anatomic models for 3D printing: application in the validation of 3D-printable models of maxillofacial bone from reduced radiation dose CT images. 3D Print Med. 2015;1:2.

Flohr TG, Schoepf UJ, Ohnesorge BM. Chasing the heart: new developments for cardiac CT. J Thorac Imaging. 2007;22:4–16.

Friedman T, Michalski M, Goodman TR, Brown JE. 3D printing from diagnostic images: a radiologist's primer with an emphasis on musculoskeletal imaging-putting the 3D printing of pathology into the hands of every physician. Skeletal Radiol. 2016;45:307–21.

Frolich AM, Spallek J, Brehmer L, Buhk JH, Krause D, Fiehler J, Kemmling A. 3D printing of intracranial aneurysms using fused deposition modeling offers highly accurate replications. AJNR Am J Neuroradiol. 2016;37:120–4.

Giannopoulos AA, Chepelev L, Sheikh A, Wang A, Dang W, Akyuz E, Hong C, Wake N, Pietila T, Dydynski PB, Mitsouras D, Rybicki FJ. 3D printed ventricular septal defect patch: a primer for the 2015 Radiological Society of North America (RSNA) hands-on course in 3D printing. 3D Print Med. 2015;1:3.

Giannopoulos AA, Steigner ML, George E, Barile M, Hunsaker AR, Rybicki FJ, Mitsouras D. Cardiothoracic applications of 3-dimensional printing. J Thorac Imaging. 2016;31(5):253–72.

Gosnell J, Pietila T, Samuel BP, Kurup HK, Haw MP, Vettukattil JJ. Integration of computed tomography and three-dimensional echocardiography for hybrid three-dimensional printing in congenital heart disease. J Digit Imaging. 2016;29(6):665–9.

Greil GF, Wolf I, Kuettner A, Fenchel M, Miller S, Martirosian P, Schick F, Oppitz M, Meinzer HP, Sieverding L. Stereolithographic reproduction of complex cardiac morphology based on high spatial resolution imaging. Clin Res Cardiol. 2007;96: 176–85.

Harrysson OL, Hosni YA, Nayfeh JF. Custom-designed orthopedic implants evaluated using finite element analysis of patient-specific computed tomography data: femoral-component case study. BMC Musculoskelet Disord. 2007;8:91.

Huang Y, Leu MC. NSF additive manufacturing workshop report. NSF Workshop on Frontiers of additive manufacturing research and education. Arlington, VA: University of Florida Center for Manufacturing Innovation; 2013.

Ionita CN, Suri H, Nataranjian S, Siddiqui A, Levy E, Hopkins NL, Bednarek DR, Rudin S. Angiographic imaging evaluation of patient-specific bifurcation-aneurysm phantom treatment with pre-shaped, self-expanding, flow-diverting stents: feasibility study. Proc SPIE. 2011;7965:79651H-1-79651H-9.

Jacobs S, Grunert R, Mohr FW, Falk V. 3D-Imaging of cardiac structures using 3D heart models for planning in heart surgery: a preliminary study. Interact Cardiovasc Thorac Surg. 2008;7:6–9.

Kozakiewicz M, Elgalal M, Loba P, Komunski P, Arkuszewski P, Broniarczyk-Loba A, Stefanczyk L. Clinical application of 3D pre-bent titanium implants for orbital floor fractures. J Craniomaxillofac Surg. 2009;37:229–34.

Mahmood F, Owais K, Taylor C, Montealegre-Gallegos M, Manning W, Matyal R, Khabbaz KR. Three-dimensional printing of mitral valve using echocardiographic data. JACC Cardiovasc Imaging. 2015;8:227–9.

Matsumoto JS, Morris JM, Foley TA, Williamson EE, Leng S, Mcgee KP, Kuhlmann JL, Nesberg LE, Vrtiska TJ. Three-dimensional physical modeling: applications and experience at Mayo Clinic. Radiographics. 2015;35:1989–2006.

Mitsouras D, Liacouras P, Imandzadeh A, Giannopoulos A, Cai T, Kumamaru K, George E, Wake N, Pomahac B, Ho V, Grant G, Rybicki F. Medical 3D printing for the radiologist. Radiographics. 2015;35(7):1965–88.

Olivieri LJ, et al. Three-dimensional printing of intracardiac defects from three-dimensional echocardiographic images: feasibility and relative accuracy. J Am Soc Echocardiogr. 2015;28(4):392–7.

Poterucha JT, Foley TA, Taggart NW. Percutaneous pulmonary valve implantation in a native outflow tract: 3-dimensional DynaCT rotational angiographic reconstruction and 3-dimensional printed model. JACC Cardiovasc Interv. 2014;7:e151–2.

Schmauss D, Haeberle S, Hagl C, Sodian R. Three-dimensional printing in cardiac surgery and interventional cardiology: a single-centre experience. Eur J Cardiothorac Surg. 2015;47:1044–52.

Tandon A, Byrne N, Nieves Velasco Forte ML, Zhang S, Dyer AK, Dillenbeck JM, Greil GF, Hussain T. Use of a semi-automated cardiac segmentation tool improves reproducibility and speed of segmentation of contaminated right heart magnetic resonance angiography. Int J Cardiovasc Imaging. 2016;32(8):1273–9.

Yoo S, Thabit O, Kim E, Ide H, Dragulescu A, Seed M, Grosse-Wortmann L, Van Arsdell G. 3D printing in medicine of congenital heart diseases. 3D Print Med. 2016;2:3.

4

Beginning and Developing a Radiology-Based In-Hospital 3D Printing Lab

Adnan Sheikh, Leonid Chepelev, Andrew M. Christensen, Dimitris Mitsouras, Betty Anne Schwarz, and Frank J. Rybicki

The number of in-hospital labs is now growing, and many reside within a radiology department. These labs are an extension of a traditional "3D visualization" lab where advanced image post-processing is routinely performed. With the advent of thin client solutions for 3D visualization, the need for a conventional 3D lab as dedicated space in a radiology department has diminished. Specifically, post-processing software to generate outputs such as multiplanar reformatted imaging and volume rendering have been integrated into and launched from PACS.

3D printing has brought new attention to 3D labs among individuals with similar interests, and like the early 3D labs within academic radiology departments, the 3D printing lab is a balance where on one side rests benefits and clinical needs and on the other side the cost and expertise. There are some differences, however, between early 3D visualization and early 3D printing. The most important difference is how an individual can enter the field. The practical reality is that the majority of 3D printing programs start with a basic fused deposition modeling (FDM) printer (Fig. 4.1). Because the cost barriers for 3D printing with this format of printing have been greatly reduced, it is often the case that a lab's first hardware (i.e., the 3D printer itself) is purchased by an individual. We are highly supportive of this practice, since a great amount of learning can be done at low cost. Many university environments now support 3D labs for students (e.g., engineering students) and other university members. While these groups function outside of the medical domain, when hospital/university campuses are centrally located, it is possible for medical practitioners to design models and then have them printed nearby. Regarding space in a hospital, or in particular a radiology department, with the lower cost of tabletop printers, a 3D lab can begin within a medical staff office or an adjacent hallway with a nearby sink. Cleaning models of their support materials requires work and space, and a comfortable environment to do these tasks, with access to a sink a waste disposal, is important for workflow.

3D printing requires that medical images, typically in DICOM format, be converted to an

A. Sheikh, M.D. (✉) • L. Chepelev, M.D.
Department of Radiology, Faculty of Medicine,
The Ottawa Hospital Research Institute,
The University of Ottawa, Ottawa, ON, Canada
e-mail: asheikh@toh.ca; lchepelev@toh.ca

A.M. Christensen
SOMADEN LLC, 8156 S. Wadsworth Blvd.,
Unit E-357, Littleton, CO 80128, USA

D. Mitsouras, Ph.D.
Applied Imaging Science Lab, Department of
Radiology, Brigham and Women's Hospital, Harvard
Medical School, Boston, MA, USA
e-mail: dmitsouras@alum.mit.edu

B.A. Schwarz, Ph.D. • F.J. Rybicki, M.D., Ph.D.
Department of Radiology, Faculty of Medicine, The
Ottawa Hospital Research Institute, The University of
Ottawa, Ottawa, ON, Canada
e-mail: frybicki@toh.ca

© Springer International Publishing AG 2017
F.J. Rybicki, G.T. Grant (eds.), *3D Printing in Medicine*, DOI 10.1007/978-3-319-61924-8_4

Fig. 4.1 3D printer managed and operated in the medical library by the medical students at the University of Ottawa, Ontario, Canada. Shown from *left* to *right*, Aili Wang, Isabelle Castonguay, Dr. Ali Jalali (physician lead), Geneviève Morin and Talia Chung in the Health Sciences Library, University of Ottawa Faculty of Medicine (Photo: Dave Weatherall, used with permission)

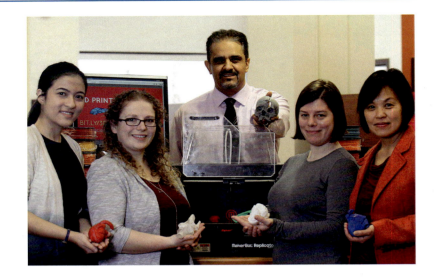

output recognized by the 3D printer. The most common output is the Standard Tessellation Language (STL) format. This material has been covered in Chap. 3 and is also described in a review article from Mitsouras et al. (2015).

Mitsouras' paper is designed as an easy-to-read treatise that is also available as a freely downloadable article. The annual meeting of the Radiological Society of North America has had several hands-on 3D printing courses; two of these have comprehensive step-by-step guides to 3D printing software that are also available as free downloads from *3D Printing in Medicine* (Chepelev et al. 2016; Giannopoulos et al. 2015). The ensemble of these three articles and Chap. 3 will provide the reader with a sound foundation of methods and software manipulations typically encountered when using a medical image to make a handheld model.

As the program grows, it is important to establish key stakeholders centered on the patient. While this chapter is written from the perspective of physician leads, leadership can come from engineers and physicists with knowledge of the anatomy. As noted earlier, the referring clinicians who perform interventions must form a partnership with technical experts (whether they be physicians or engineers), and there is a large role for radiology technologists, other individuals to perform segmentation, individuals that include students to operate the printers and clean/prepare

the models, and a specific individual to take the role as quality lead.

Segmentation requires experience and a meticulous approach and can be performed by physicians and technologists. While most models are generated from either CT or MRI, cases may require co-registration if both modalities are required to delineate specific pathology. While the typical diagnostic images are frequently usable for segmentation, repeated studies with external patient markers and specific volumetric sequences in the case of MRI or thin axial slices in the case of CT imaging may be needed. While it is not desirable, particularly in children and young adults, repeating an imaging study is sometimes the best pathway to optimum care to ensure segmentation accuracy, based on the spatial resolution needed, or the mitigation of artifacts in the initial images.

Once the lab includes a larger-format printer, the device itself requires engineering support; this will ensure adequate functioning, including regular maintenance and rigorous quality assurance to ensure prints that adhere to institution- and disease-specific error tolerance thresholds. While quality assurance is discussed in detail below, specific quality guidelines have not been established. However, recommendations are now emerging from societies such as the RSNA Special Interest Group to enhance quality of 3D models. In practice, tolerance thresholds for model accuracy are typically established upon discussion with the radiologists and interventionalists with specific disease pathophysiology and patient in mind. For example, a tumor with a 20 mm resection margin with no neurological involvement may be subject to less stringent criteria than an intracranial intraparenchymal mass in close proximity to major vasculature. Regardless of the accepted tolerance threshold and 3DP technology, regular maintenance and vigilant quality assurance are indispensable in ensuring 3DP program success.

As the lab progresses, undoubtedly the service line will receive requests to make more complicated models and to make changes to the anatomy (e.g., mirroring one side of the face) when helping to plan complex interventions. Thus, when formulating the hardware and software requirements for the lab, we present the following perspective for the common applications for medical 3D printing. These follow the outline from Christensen and Rybicki (2017), we have found that the most useful method to categorize the applications is by the intended use:

Group I. **Anatomical Models**. A model representing as-scanned anatomy. The intended use for anatomic models is procedural planning and/or a reference during the procedure, for education including simulation and for informed consent. The defining characteristic of Group I models is that what is printed is intended to exactly reproduce the anatomy captured by the medical imaging device.

Group II. **Modified Anatomical Models**. A modified model of anatomy, simple surgical planning performed digitally to further enhance the model, significantly modified models. For Group II models, the intended use is enhanced surgical planning and guidance, but unlike Group I models, the anatomy being held in the end users hand is purposely modified from the patient anatomy.

Group III. **Virtual Surgical Planning with Templates**. This group refers to complex surgical planning done digitally, for example, 3D-printed templates/models/guides produced which are intended to guide the digital

plan on the patient in the operating room. The intended use for Group III models is to augment the surgical procedure with specific pre-planned steps which are carried out in surgery using 3D-printed guides or templates.

These three groups are also used to organize workflow, elaborate on post-processing, and to put into framework important regulatory considerations. A common "first model" or experimental scenario begins with a CT scan of bone that is used to design Group I models, printed on a single-spool FDM printer. The CT scan undergoes 3D visualization using tools that are familiar to the radiologist. However, since these tools often do not have STL output or have an STL output that requires additional modifications before printing, out the outset, freeware for computer-aided design (CAD) is typically used to generate a printable STL file. The bone is very amenable to thresholding methods from noncontrast CT scans, simplifying the process of 3D printing.

While the barriers for a rudimentary 3DP program are relatively low, success is predicated upon clinical applications. One highly useful, early strategy for a developing in-hospital 3D printing lab is partnership between radiologists and one group of specialist physicians. Within that specialty, complex cases frequently require detailed discussions, supported by precise measurements of anatomical relationships as well as consideration of disease pathophysiology. The radiologist often prepares 3D visualization to augment these conversations, and very often 3D printing can further clarify complex anatomy. For example, in a relationship with orthopedic surgeons, specific models of bone tumors of the pelvis will prove useful to delineate surgical planes and help foster a relationship and confidence in the models for procedure planning.

A logical next step for a growing 3D printing lab is to add a second, relatively low budget vat polymerization system. With these systems, the scope of models will increase, and a modest-sized build tray will not be prohibitively expensive (Fig. 4.2). The acquisition of a vat polymerization system certainly could come

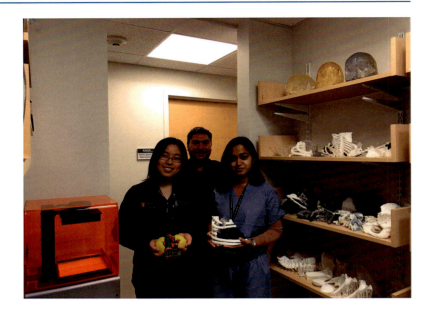

Fig. 4.2 3D Printing at the Applied Imaging Science Laboratory, Boston, MA. From *left* to *right*: Anji Tang, Dimitrios Mitsouras PhD, Elizabeth George, MD

before a FDM printer, but by the time both are in the lab, additional human resources will be necessary to manage the printers, clean the models, and manage orders from referring clinicians. With these experiences in hand, larger printers should then be considered, and with this comes a wide scope of services and collaborations within the institution and beyond. At present, there are a limited number of hospitals with advanced resources, making them desirable for partnerships as medical 3D printing continues its exponential growth.

Typically derived from CT or MRI, Group I 3D models are designed to depict the anatomic information contained in the medical images, without alteration, and are generally used for surgical planning. Examples include a newborn with double outlet right ventricle (Medical Modeling 2012) or craniomaxillofacial models where tissues are not altered, for example, to plan complex procedures including congenital deformity corrections and secondary reconstruction following trauma (D'Urso et al. 1999; Yoo et al. 2015; Christensen et al. 2004). Orthopedic (Brown et al. 2003) and cardiovascular (Giannopoulos et al. 2016) applications include 3D-printed models for visualization and physical, hands-on simulation. The common denominator for Group I models is that 3D printing extends current 3D

visualization and the model does not differ from the patient's anatomy. Following the Modeling Flow Map of Christensen and Rybicki (2017), we maintain that steps A–E, including "3D Printing Preparation," should use systems (software and some hardware) that are cleared by the FDA for their intended use. This includes not only the imaging hardware/software but also the software used to segment the medical images from their original 2D state into a 3D dataset usable for 3D printing (i.e., an STL or 3MF file) (FDA 2014a, b). Regarding the steps "Build Prep—Support, Slicing" to the end of the pathway when models are used by healthcare professionals, the FDA has commented that work in hospital is not under these auspices, and they do not contain what the FDA considers to be medical devices (Yoo et al. 2015).

In this scenario, step E "3D Printing Preparation: Minor Changes" does not make significant changes to the anatomy but instead refines the STL file so that it can be printed. Since the anatomy of the printed part has been finalized in step D, these minor modifications are grouped with the later steps in the workflow of generating the model after the completion of the design. As described in Christensen and Rybicki (2017), minor modifications have the intent of not modifying the original anatomy but rather highlighting an area, labeling the model, or adding material to allow for better 3D printing production. The following are examples of minor modifications of the models:

1. Filling holes in anatomy introduced by imaging artifact
2. Smoothing anatomy in anatomical areas where imaging artifact has been introduced
3. Adding structural supports to keep anatomy in proper relation to other anatomy
4. Adding material as a "wall" around a contrast-enhanced object (such as a vessel lumen), commonly used for heart or vascular modeling
5. Removing known imaging artifact
6. Labeling the model
7. Cutting the model into parts for better visualization or 3D printability
8. Adding magnets to allow for better functionality of cut models
9. Adding color to delineate or highlight anatomical structures
10. Grouping separate anatomical structures into a single model file

We recognize that software packages may be designed to do these preparation steps as well as more major modifications spelled out in step F. However, patients who require substantial modifications to the anatomy captured in the medical images should be considered in Group II: Modified Anatomical Models.

3D-printed models that fall into Group II, noted as "Modified Anatomical Models," have the common characteristic that the anatomy as captured by the medical imaging device has been "significant" to enhance the planning of an intervention. Common examples include printing a patient's anatomy with a tumor "digitally" removed. Another common example is mirroring a patient's anatomy. These models have the same steps A–D Group I models, but patients for whom the 3D output falls into Group II include both step F (major changes) as well as E (minor changes). Examples of major modifications from Christensen and Rybicki (2017) are as follows:

1. Removal of segmented anatomy such as a tumor, in order to visualize the size of the defect before reconstruction.
2. Mirroring of the dataset to provide a mirror image model in order to ascertain degree of symmetry or asymmetry.
3. Mirroring and "perfecting" of the dataset to provide a model which appears to be "perfect" (a unilateral defect has now been erased by combining half of a mirror image model with the half of the unaffected original patient model).
4. Digital placement of a "graft" of either alloplastic or autogenous material into a defect and including this on the resultant model.
5. Visualizing, sizing, and simulating intervention using another medical device digitally and subtracting said device, its shadow, screw holes/fixation points, etc. from the original model, leaving an imprint/pattern/holes of some type on the model.
6. Visualizing, sizing, and simulating intervention using another medical device and altering the model in some way that includes this device.
7. Designing a graft of alloplastic or autogenous material and printing out the model with an indication of this graft or a printout of the new graft itself. An example includes a patient with a cranioplasty defect and filling the defect with a perfectly fitting implant template which will be used to guide harvest of autogenous material or shaping/manufacturing of alloplastic material.

We maintain that software used to make major modifications should be FDA cleared for this intended use and that printed model should also be considered a medical device. We do note, however, that 3D printing within hospitals are within the scope of medical practice, and as such in the United States, these practices are subject to regulations set by specific institutions and societies as opposed to the FDA. This places important roles and responsibilities on medical societies such as the RSNA, as noted in more detail below. Should the hospital be outsourcing models for commercial use, or if the models are generated by a company that is marketing models in Group II for patient care, the hardware (i.e., the 3D printer) and the software used to drive the hardware should be FDA cleared for these intended uses.

Group III models are denoted by Christensen and Rybicki has "Virtual Surgical Planning with Templates," typically referring to the digital process based on CT or MR images, for example, a CT scan in patient who needs reconstructive osseous surgery to the face (Gateno et al. 2007; Hirsch et al. 2009; Mardini et al. 2014). Digital surgical planning informs the design of templates and guides incorporated into patient intervention. The number of in hospital Group II models is increasing, although to achieve these goals, the most modern software (Imprint, Materialise, Leuven, Netherlands) must be combined with an advanced printer.

We opine that radiologists occupy a central and indispensable role in clinical 3DP and certainly in patients for whom models are generated from CT or MR images. Moving forward, radiologists will have to assume a deepened role in ensuring overall quality as well as managing image protocolling and acquisition, to the level of precise segmentation of disease extent and CAD of surgical guides, instruments, and implants. At present, radiologists are uniquely positioned to communicate with all involved stakeholders regarding the extent of disease, providing quality assurance for both the mathematical and the physical 3DP models and productively engaging in multidisciplinary rounds to communicate model features and limitations.

Organizations with medical specialties, for example, the RSNA or the American College of Radiology, will be charged with generating professional standards for in-hospital printing. Early adopters of medical 3D printing currently populate these groups, for example, the Special Interest Group of the RSNA. In our experience, the general rule has been that those early adopters have maintained high-quality printing, factoring in and self-regulating all of the steps that could lead to clinically significant differences between the 3D-printed model and the desired output intended for patient care. While we expect that this will be

managed by regulatory bodies, for example, the FDA and Health Canada, there is far less regulation of what can happen within the walls of a hospital. Thus, the burden is likely to fall on societies to limit risk. The most important of these risks in our opinion is "freeware" or software without proven credentials by regulatory bodies being used to post-process and alter patient DICOM datasets for medical use. Similarly, the scope of printing hardware has large boundaries, including printers for $100 USD. Groups such as the Special Interest Group are very actively working to create recommendations to ensure that quality and safety are maintained. Because this topic is so important for healthcare, we have dedicated Chap. 11 in this book to address these issues. We believe that rigor must be maintained as the next generation of medical modelers rapidly outnumbers the early adopters. We maintain the patient experience as the top priority, and accuracy as paramount to optimizing this experience, even if this decision has a higher cost to the 3D printing lab. Finally, we believe that the best results will come at the intersection of hospitals, regulatory bodies, and industry, and we encourage interactions among all three groups as 3D printing emerges as a universal tool to improve the quality of life for our patients.

References

Brown GA, et al. Rapid prototyping: the future of trauma surgery? J Bone Joint Surg Am. 2003;85(Suppl 4): 49–55.

Chepelev L, Hodgdon T, Gupta A, Wang A, Torres C, Krishna S, Akyuz E, Mitsouras D, Sheikh A. Medical 3D printing for vascular interventions and surgical oncology: a primer for the 2016 radiological society of North America (RSNA) hands-on course in 3D printing. 3D Print Med. 2016;2:5. doi:10.1186/s41205-016-0008-6.

Christensen A, Rybicki FJ. Maintaining safety and efficacy for 3D printing in medicine. 3D Print Med. 2017;3:1.

Christensen AM, et al. Advanced "tactile" medical imaging for separation surgeries of conjoined twins. Childs Nerv Syst. 2004;20(8-9):547–53.

D'Urso PS, et al. Stereolithographic biomodelling in cranio-maxillofacial surgery: a prospective trial. J Craniomaxillofac Surg. 1999;27(1):30–7.

FDA. Public Workshop - Additive manufacturing of medical devices: an interactive discussion on the technical considerations of 3D printing, October 8–9, 2014. 2014a. http://www.fda.gov/MedicalDevices/NewsEvents/WorkshopsConferences/ucm397324.htm. Accessed 16 October 2016.

FDA. Medical devices - is the product a medical device?. 2014b. http://www.fda.gov/MedicalDevices/DeviceRegulationandGuidance/Overview/ClassifyYourDevice/ucm051512.htm. Accessed 16 October 2016.

Gateno J, et al. Clinical feasibility of computer-aided surgical simulation (CASS) in the treatment of complex cranio-maxillofacial deformities. J Oral Maxillofac Surg. 2007;65(4):728–34.

Giannopoulos AA, Chepelev L, Sheikh A, Wang A, Dang W, Akyuz E, Hong C, Wake N, Pietila T, Dydynski PB, Mitsouras D, Rybicki FJ. 3D printed ventricular septal defect patch: a primer for the 2015 Radiological Society of North America (RSNA) hands-on course in 3D printing. 3D Print Med. 2015;1:3. doi:10.1186/s41205-015-0002-4.

Giannopoulos AA, Mitsouras D, Yoo SJ, Liu PP, Chatzizisis YS, Rybicki FJ. Applications of 3D printing in cardiovascular diseases. Nat Rev Cardiol. 2016;13(12):701–18. doi:10.1038/nrcardio.2016.170. Review.

Hirsch DL, et al. Use of computer-aided design and computer-aided manufacturing to produce orthognathically ideal surgical outcomes: a paradigm shift in head and neck reconstruction. J Oral Maxillofac Surg. 2009;67(10):2115–22.

Mardini S, et al. Three-dimensional preoperative virtual planning and template use for surgical correction of craniosynostosis. J Plast Reconstr Aesthet Surg. 2014;67(3):336–43.

Medical Modeling. 510(k) Summary K120956 - VSP System. 2012. http://www.accessdata.fda.gov/cdrh_docs/pdf12/K120956.pdf. Accessed 16 October 2016.

Mitsouras D, Liacouras P, Imanzadeh A, Giannopoulos AA, Cai T, Kumamaru KK, George E, Wake N, Caterson EJ, Pomahac B, Ho VB, Grant GT, Rybicki FJ. Medical 3D printing for the radiologist. Radiographics. 2015;35(7):23.

Yoo S-J, et al. 3D printing in medicine of congenital heart diseases. 3D Print Med. 2015;2(1):3.

Craniofacial Applications of 3D Printing

5

Gerald T. Grant and Peter C. Liacouras

Current advances in imaging technology, virtual surgical planning, and 3D printing have potentially changed how we will use patient-specific information for treatment planning and customized treatment. Medical providers can not only view a 3D rendering of the patient's anatomy on digital display, but that image can now be transferred as a physical model which not only aids in treatment planning but in patient education. The use of these technologies in craniofacial reconstruction was reported in the early 1990s (Gronet et al. 2003). These techniques have proven to provide surgeons confidence in executing their plan, reduced operating times, and better outcomes. In addition, they provide patient-centered care and better esthetic and functional outcomes (Grant et al. 2013) (Fig. 5.1). In this chapter, we will review some of the areas of application in craniofacial reconstruction and dentistry.

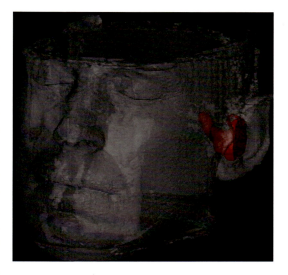

Fig. 5.1 Identification of the auditory canal from a cone beam CT

G.T. Grant, D.M.D., M.S. (✉)
Oral Health and Rehabilitation, University of Louisville, School of Dentistry, Louisville, KY, USA
e-mail: gerald.grant@louisville.edu

P.C. Liacouras, Ph.D.
Department of Radiology, 3D Medical Applications Center, Walter Reed National Military Medical Center (WRNMMC), Bldg 1, Rm 4417B, 8901 Wisconsin Avenue, Bethesda, MD 20889, USA
e-mail: peter.c.liacouras.civ@mail.mil

5.1   Craniofacial Imaging

Computed tomography is the preferred method of imaging for head and neck reconstructions. The Hounsfield scale enables identification of soft and hard tissues by their density; this allows for segmentation of the images for reconstruction of 3D models with minimal artifact but at the expense of radiation exposure to the patient (Gordon et al. 2014). In contrast, cone beam computed tomography (CBCT) has become more common in dental and medical practices; their low radiation exposure provides a unique opportunity to capture hard tissue

© Springer International Publishing AG 2017
F.J. Rybicki, G.T. Grant (eds.), *3D Printing in Medicine*, DOI 10.1007/978-3-319-61924-8_5

images that have been used for endodontic diagnosis, airway visualization, orthognathic reconstructions, and dental implant planning (Gronet et al. 2003; Vannier 2003; Grant et al. 2013; Estrela et al. 2008). However, CBCT is subject to severe artifact from dental restorations, and lack the contrast to segment soft tissue to complement bone. In addition, due to the inconsistancy of contrast, the Hounsfield Scale does not apply to identify soft versus bone tissues.

Surface scanning has also been used to design and fabricate craniofacial devices. These are non-invasive and have applications in craniofacial planning (Sabol and Grant 2011). These scanning devices use laser, light, or some type of contact scanning technologies employing technologies such as stereo photogrammetry to increase accuracy, and are stationary or handheld (Knoops et al. 2017). The images captured are often used for registration to other medical images to provide more accurate virtual models for virtual planning and to design devices, medical models,

and surgical guides. In addition, surface scanning has also been successfully used to fabricate maxillofacial prostheses (Sabol and Grant 2011; Grant et al. 2015).

5.2 Cranioplasty

Cranial defects can be caused by trauma, tumor, or decompressive craniotomy. Historically, the fabrication of a custom cranial implant involved an ambulatory patient, conventional impression techniques, fabricating an indirect stone model of the defect, and fabricating a mold for processing polymethyl methacrylate (PMMA) (Aquilino et al. 1988). Surgical placement involved extensive modification to get an acceptable fit with long hours in the operating room and use of self-curing acrylics to fill in the gaps. The initial use of 3D printing was to print the defect from which a custom wax implant could be fabricated and a mold for PMMA (Fig. 5.2). In this process, the

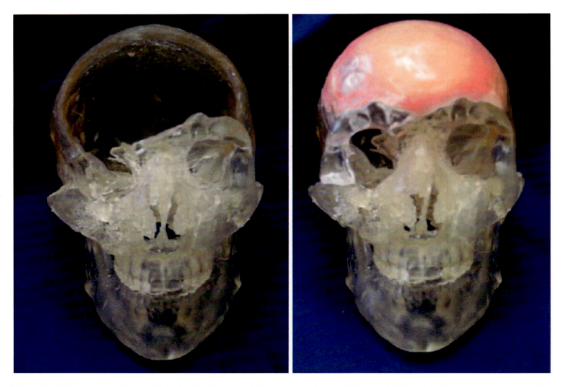

Fig. 5.2 The *left* photo is the SLA skull with a frontal bone and lateral orbit defect. The *right* is the waxed implant for mold fabrication

patient does not have to be available to the laboratory, and the process enables more complicated craniofacial implants that fit the defect with minimal modification, cutting the fabrication time down by close to 75%, and operating time nearly in half (Gronet et al. 2003) (Fig. 5.2). This process has now evolved to digital design directly from medical imaging and fabrication of the cranial implant by milling PMMA and Polyetheretherketone (PEEK) implants or 3D-printed titanium and Polyethyl ketone ketone (PEKK) (Fig. 5.3).

5.3   Craniofacial Reconstruction

In trauma cases, 3D models may help to recognize the position and the direction of fractures, the number of bone fragments, and the degree of dislocation. Virtual planning can assist in a reconstruction plan with reestablishing contours and fabricating positioning and bending guides for plates and recontour bars. However, there are limitations that can result in surgical delay due to long model production with current additive manufacturing processes (Powers et al. 1998; Holck et al. 1999; McAllister 1998) (Fig. 5.4).

Virtual simulation and printed models from medical images provide solid models that simulate osteotomies and grafts, simulate segmental jaw movements, and facilitate preoperative

construction of surgical guides, templates, and custom surgical devices (Ander et al. 1994; D'Urso et al. 1999; Kermer et al. 1998).

Guides can be designed and fabricated that allow the prebending of recontouring bars for mandibular stabilization prior to the surgical reduction, positioning guides that reapproximate bone sections for plating, cutting guides to move bone as needed, and customized devices to replace or stabilize sections of the mandible, zygoma, or orbit using biocompatible materials (Singarea et al. 2004). Using virtual surgical techniques, the surgical guides assist the surgeon in osteotomy cuts, implant placement, positioning of bone and soft tissue for reconstruction, and assistance in prebending of reconstruction plates (Fig. 5.5).

Recently, the limits of craniofacial reconstruction have been challenged with the success of full total face transplants. The same principles of virtual planning can be very useful in the selection of appropriate anatomical donors to approximate the correct dental occlusion and other anatomical reconstructions. (Murphy et al. 2015a; Sosin et al. 2016) (Fig. 5.6). Cutting guides can be designed to provide an intimate fit of bone margins of the donor anatomy to the recipient site. Current research in this area proposes navigational

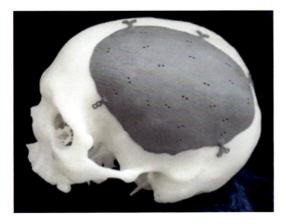

Fig. 5.3 Titanium cranial implant manufactured directly from electron beam melting

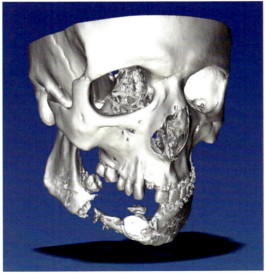

Fig. 5.4 3D rendering of defect of the mandible

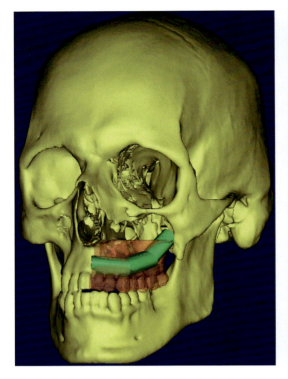

Fig. 5.5 Virtual planning for a fibula reconstruction of the maxilla

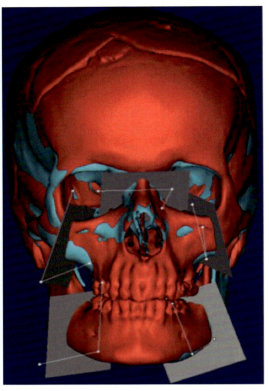

Fig. 5.6 Both the donor and the recipient skulls have been registered and cutting planes established to fabricate cutting guides

technologies and mastication simulation (Gordon et al. 2014; Murphy et al. 2015b).

In respect to the donors, a facial mask is required after the harvest of the transplant. Conventional fabrication of a total facial prostheses by a maxillofacial prosthodontist or anaplastologist at the time of the surgery can be disruptive and expensive. An alternative technique using 3D printing from medical imaging and photographs have been proposed, as they can be fabricated directly or with a mold, prior to the surgical intervention at a lower cost (Grant et al. 2014) (Fig. 5.7).

5.4 Dental Implant Guides

Dental implant placement is driven by the restorative plan it retains or supports. The purpose of a surgical guide is to assist the surgeon in the location and direction of the osteotomy prior to dental implant placement. The Academy of Prosthodontics

defines a surgical template as a guide used to assist in proper surgical placement and angulations of dental implants (The Glossary of Prosthodontic Terms, 2017). Based on the amount of the operative restriction of the drill, the design of the surgical template can be classified as nonrestrictive, partially restrictive, or completely restrictive (Stumpel 2008; Misch and Dietsh-Misch 1999). Historically, surgical guides were fabricated conventionally on dental casts using a variety of techniques and materials including clear vacuum-formed matrix, freeform auto-polymerizing acrylic resin and acrylic resin duplicates of the available prosthesis or diagnostic wax-ups.

Recently, software has become more available that provides dental implant planning from CBCT using digital scans of diagnostic wax-ups or virtual restorations from intraoral scans or diagnostic casts. By registering the images, the restoration can be planned, and a surgical guide

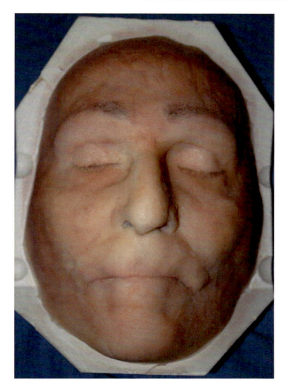

Fig. 5.7 Silicone-fabricated donor mask for donor of facial transplant. Fabricated prior to the transplant surgery

can be fabricated to limit the placement of the dental implant to accommodate the restorative plan (Fig. 5.8). In some instances, this workflow allows for "same day" implant retained restorations, even in more complicated cases requiring grafting (Cheng et al. 2008; Stapleton et al. 2014). Once the digital or virtual plans have been designed, the guides and the restorations can be produced with digital manufacturing—either additive or milled.

Most additive manufacturing technologies can be used to fabricate the surgical guides; however, there are some concerns of irritation from residual surface chemicals of some polymers. USP (US Pharmacopeia) Class VI judges the suitability of plastic material intended for use as containers or accessories for parenteral preparations. Suitability under USP Class VI is typically a base requirement for medical device manufacturers. It is recommended that materials compliant with this test be used for all surgical guides as well as medical/dental models available in a surgical setting. Most manufacturers of 3D printers will have a medical grade material that is Class VI compliant and offer a specific

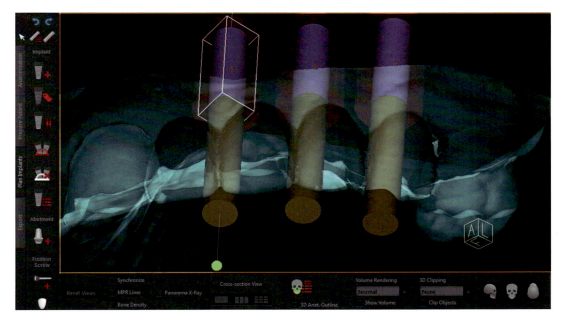

Fig. 5.8 Dental implant placement based on digitally designed restorative solution. The teeth are replaced "digitally" and angulation and depth of implants are determined to manufacture an implant placement guide

cleaning process for these items. However, the Food and Drug Administration (FDA) has cleared devices for surgical guides and limited intraoral use produced by 3D printed materials (Formlabs, Cambridge, MA), and it is expected that there may be similar trends in the future. This is further detailed in Chap. 10.

5.5 Maxillofacial Prosthetics

Trained maxillofacial prosthodontists along with technicians or anaplastologists have historically achieved the planning and fabrication of facial features through moulage and sculpting techniques. These techniques are usually uncomfortable to the patient and require several days to fabricate the prosthesis. In contrast, medical images provide the information that will allow for virtual planning and fabrication of facial prostheses. Software mirroring techniques can be used to "sculpt" missing ears or missing anatomy on the contralateral side and software that provides "electronic clay" type technologies (Geomagics Freeform, 3D Systems) allow for development of textures, accommodate attachments, and design molds for CAD/CAM or 3D printing (Jiao et al. 2004; Liacouras et al. 2011). Molds are then layered and colored with silicone since currently there are no commercial silicone printers that would allow for direct fabrication and color (Fig. 5.9). Recent advancements in lower-priced scanners and online maxillofacial design commercial sites are making these technologies more accessible to providers outside academic and military practices.

5.6 Other Craniofacial Applications

Aside from reconstruction and dental applications, benign tumors of the jaw usually present with localized expanding deformities. Other pathology and vascular lesions can be differentiated with contrast enhanced CT. Printed models provide vital information for planning and patient education, offering a physical model of the affected area (Fig. 5.10). In addition, using virtual surgical planning with a color-coding technique, specific structures such as teeth, nerves, and the extent of a tumor can be displayed, facilitating more detailed surgical planning (Santler et al. 1998).

Forensic reconstruction is another area of application of digital planning and 3D printing. An unpublished work by the Naval Postgraduate Dental School's Craniofacial lab working with the Exploited Children's section of the FBI validated soft tissue reconstruction software from CT images of complete and incomplete skulls (Fig. 5.11), suggesting that computer reconstruction can be valuable in skull reconstructions historically done by forensic artists.

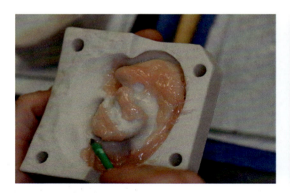

Fig. 5.9 Additive manufactured ear mold being layered with colored silicone

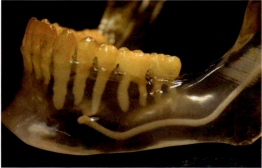

Fig. 5.10 3D printed model of a mandible with teeth and lingual nerve highlighted with different colors

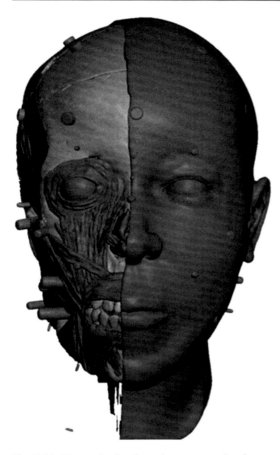

Fig. 5.11 Electronic clay forensic reconstruction from a skull

5.7 Conclusions

Continual advances in medical imaging, reconstruction software, and 3D printing continue to aid and advance the field of craniofacial surgery and other medical specialties. Technology advances, including more user-friendly software will enhance utlization. As these technologies become increasingly available and affordable, adoption may eventually become routine.

References

Ander H, Zur Nedden D, Muhlbauer W. CT-guided stereolithography as a new tool in craniofacial surgery. Br J Plast Surg. 1994;47:60–4.

Aquilino SA, Jordan RD, White JT. Fabrication of an alloplastic implant for the cranial implant. J Prosthet Dent. 1988;59(1):68–71.

Cheng AC, Tee-Khin N, Siew-Luen C, Lee H, Wee AG. The management of a severely resorbed edentulous maxilla using a bone graft and a CAD/CAM-guided immediately loaded definitive implant prosthesis: a clinical report. J Prosthet Dent. 2008;99(2):85–90.

D'Urso PS, Barker TM, Earwaker WJ, Bruce LJ, Atkinson RL, Lanigan MW, Arvier JF, Effeney DJ. Stereolithography biomodelling in craniomaxillofacial surgery: a prospective trial. J Craniomaxillofac Surg. 1999;27:30–7.

Estrela C, Bueno MR, Azevedo BC, Azevedo JR, Pécora JD. A new periapical index based on cone beam computed tomography. J Endod. 2008; 34(11):1325–31.

Glossary of Prosthodontic Terms: ninth edition. 2017 May;117(5S):e1-e105.

Gordon CR, Murphy RJ, Coon D, Basafa E, Otake Y, Al Rakan M, Rada E, Susarla S, Swanson E, Fishman E, Santiago G, Brandacher G, Liacouras P, Grant G, Armand M. Preliminary development of a workstation for craniomaxillofacial surgical procedures: introducing a computer-assisted planning and execution system. J Craniofac Surg. 2014;25(1):273–83.

Grant GT, Liacouras P, Santiago G, Garcia JR, Al Rakan M, Murphy R, Armand M, Gordon CR. Restoration of the donor face after facial allotransplantation: digital manufacturing techniques. Ann Plast Surg. 2014;72(6):720–4.

Grant GT, Kondor S, Liacouras P. Maxillofacial imaging in the trauma patient. Atlas Oral Maxillofac Surg Clin North Am. 2013;21(1):25–36.

Grant GT, Liacouras P, Aitaholmes C, Garnes J, Wilson WO. Digital capture, design, and manufacturing of a facial prosthesis: clinical report of a pediatric patient. J Prosthet Dent. 2015;114(1):138–41.

Gronet PM, Waskewicz GA, Richardson C. Preformed Acrylic Cranial Implants using fused deposition modeling: a clinical report. J Prosthet Dent. 2003;90(5):429–33.

Holck DEE, Boyd EM Jr, Ng J, Mauffray RO. Benefits of stereolithography in orbital reconstruction. Ophthalmology. 1999;106:1214–8.

Jiao T, Zhang F, Huang X, Wang C. Design and fabrication of auricular prostheses by CAD/CAM system. Int J Prosthodont. 2004;17:460–3.

Kermer C, Rasse M, Lagogiannis G, Undt G, Wagner A, Millesi W. Colour stereolithography for planning complex maxillofacial tumour surgery. J Craniomaxillofac Surg. 1998;26:360–2.

Knoops PG, Beaumont CA, Borghi A, Rodriguez-Florez N, Breakey RW, Rodgers W, Angullia F, Jeelani NU, Schievano S, Dunaway DJ. Comparison of three-dimensional scanner systems for craniomaxillofacial imaging. J Plast Reconstr Aesthet Surg. 2017;70(4):441–9.

Liacouras P, Garnes J, Roman R, Grant GT. Auricular prosthetic design and manufacturing using computed tomography, 3D photographic imaging and rapid prototyping. J Prosthet Dent. 2011;105(2):80–2.

McAllister ML. Application of stereolithography to subperiosteal implants manufacture. J Oral Implantol. 1998;24:89–92.

Misch CE, Dietsh-Misch F. Diagnostic casts, preimplant prosthodontics, treatment prostheses, and surgical templates. In: Misch CE, editor. Contemporary implant dentistry. 2nd ed. St Louis, MO: Mosby; 1999. p. 135–50.

Murphy RJ, Gordon CR, Basafa E, Liacouras P, Grant GT, Armand M. Computer-assisted, Le Fort-based, face-jaw-teeth transplantation: a pilot study on system feasibility and translational assessment. Int J Comput Assist Radiol Surg. 2015b;10(7):1117–26.

Murphy RJ, Basafa E, Hashemi S, Grant GT, Liacouras P, Susarla SM, Otake Y, Santiago G, Armand M, Gordon CR. Optimizing hybrid occlusion in face-jaw-teeth transplantation: a preliminary assessment of real-time cephalometery as part of the computer-assisted planning and execution workstation for crani-omaxillofacial surgery. Plast Reconstr Surg. 2015a;136(2):350–62.

Powers DB, Edgin WA, Tabatchnick L. Stereolithography: a historical review and indications or use in the management of trauma. J Craniomaxillofac Trauma. 1998;4:16–23.

Sabol J, Grant GT. Digital image capture and rapid prototyping of the maxillofacial defect. J Prosthodont. 2011;20(4):310–4.

Santler G, Kärcher H, Ruda C. Indications and limitations of three-dimensional models in craniomaxillofacial surgery. J Craniomaxillofac Surg. 1998;26:11–6.

Singarea S, Dichena L, Lu B, Yanpub L, Zhenyub G, Yaxionga L. Design and fabrication of custom mandible titanium tray based on rapid prototyping. Med Eng Phys. 2004;26(8):671–6.

Sosin M, Ceradini DJ, Hazen A, Levine JP, Staffenberg DA, Saadeh PB, Flores RL, Brecht LE, Bernstein GL, Rodriguez ED. Total face, eyelids, ears, scalp, and skeletal subunit transplant cadaver simulation: the culmination of aesthetic, craniofacial, and microsurgery principles. Plast Reconstr Surg. 2016;137(5):1569–81.

Stapleton BM, Lin WS, Ntounis A, Harris BT, Morton D. Application of digital diagnostic impression, virtual planning, and computer-guided implant surgery for a CAD/CAM-fabricated, implant-supported fixed dental prosthesis: a clinical report. J Prosthet Dent. 2014;112(3):402–8.

Stumpel LJ 3rd. Cast-based guided implant placement: a novel technique. J Prosthet Dent. 2008;100:61–9.

Vannier MW. Craniofacial computed tomography scanning: technology applications and future trends. Orthod Craniofac Res. 2003;6(Suppl. 1):23–30.

3D Printing in Neurosurgery

6

Vicknes Waran, Vairavan Narayanan,
Ravindran Karrupiah, and Chun Yoong Cham

6.1   Introduction

3D printing is generating interest in many fields, for example, design, engineering, and medicine. The surgical fields in medicine have taken the lead in progress, especially in orthopedics, maxillofacial reconstruction, and neurosurgery (Eltorai et al. 2015; Yang et al. 2015; Mavili et al. 2007; Müller et al. 2003; McGurk et al. 1997). In particular, 3D printing has contributed greatly to the development of personalized medicine. 3D printing has emerged to play a unique role in the fabrication of personalized implants as well as in surgical planning and simulation, assisting in the consent process, and providing an educational tool for medical students and residents (Mavili et al. 2007; Müller et al. 2003; McGurk et al. 1997; Liew et al. 2015; Jones et al. 2016; Naftulin et al. 2015; Rengier et al. 2010; Webb 2000). This is based on the fact that reasonably complex 3D-printed models can be created in a short period of time with a good cost efficiency.

6.2   Neurosurgery

The application of 3D printing in the field of neurosurgery began in 2007 when researchers started developing implants and plates to reconstruct facial bones and skull defects (Kozakiewicz et al. 2009; Klammert et al. 2010; Li et al. 2013; Zhang et al. 2014). This was an appropriate starting point, as commercially available printers were still in their infancy and only allowed printing in single material and density.

3D printing progressed, following the evidence that models were accurate spatial representations of patient anatomy. By 2012, printers that were able to print in more than one material and density (Shore value) were available. The advent of these new printers allowed researchers and clinicians to create lifelike, spatially, and anatomically accurate models that could be used in the training of surgeons, patient understanding,

Electronic Supplementary Material The online version of this chapter (doi:10.1007/978-3-319-61924-8_6) contains supplementary material, which is available to authorized users.

V. Waran, F.R.C.S. (Neurosurg) (✉)
Department of Surgery, University of Malaya, Kuala Lumpur, Malaysia

University of Malaya Specialist Centre, Kuala Lumpur, Malaysia

Centre for Biomedical and Technology Integration (CBMTI), Kuala Lumpur, Malaysia
e-mail: cmvwaran@gmail.com; cmvwaran@um.edu.my

V. Narayanan, F.R.C.S. (Neurosurg) • R. Karrupiah, M.S. (Surg) • C.Y. Cham, M.B.B.S.
Centre for Biomedical and Technology Integration (CBMTI), Kuala Lumpur, Malaysia

F.J. Rybicki, G.T. Grant (eds.), *3D Printing in Medicine*, DOI 10.1007/978-3-319-61924-8_6

and planning of complex procedures (Narayanan et al. 2015; Tai et al. 2015; Zheng et al. 2016; Ploch et al. 2016).

The aim of this chapter is to trace these developments, the use of the end products, challenges encountered, and future application possibilities.

6.3   Cranial and Facial Implants

In neurosurgery, the initial application of 3D printing technology can be traced to maxillofacial procedures where surgeons reconstructed and or repair of facial and calvarial defects, usually secondary to developmental, traumatic, or postsurgical defects (Solaro et al. 2008; Winder et al. 1999; Dean et al. 2003; Rotaru et al. 2012). The geometry of the facial bones and skull being extremely complex, it is often a challenge to mold plates to accurately fit and provide suitable cosmetic reconstruction (Caro-Osorio et al. 2013; Marbacher et al. 2012; Fathi et al. 2008). Since most of these defects primarily involve underlying bony structures, the application of this technology proved ideal.

Computer-generated images were also used to reconstruct bony defects from a composite using the normal opposite side. This "mirroring," now commonly used in models that fall in the category of "modified anatomical models," (Christensen and Rybicki 2017) is not always possible as patients often had bilateral defects. Therefore computer algorithms to mirror or reconstruct from scratch was required. Initial plates used were hand-molded, based on computer graphics (Caro-Osorio et al. 2013; Marbacher et al. 2012; Fathi et al. 2008; Shah et al. 2014).

With the advent of 3D printing, models were initially created in the corrected form, and titanium plates were molded to fit the defect based on the reconstruction. The reconstructed plates were tested on the defect model prior to sterilization and surgery (Solaro et al. 2008; Winder et al. 1999; Dean et al. 2003; Rotaru et al. 2012; D'Urso et al. 2000).

Based on the initial experience learned above, the use of 3D printing for neurosurgical applications was extended to replacing cranial defects. This represented a large need in neurosurgery, as patients often have large segments of their skull removed following severe head injuries as means of controlling rises in intracranial pressure.

Historically, cranial reconstructions were carried out by using the autologous calvarial bone that is removed from the patient during initial surgery and stored in the abdomen of the patient or freeze dried (Shah et al. 2014; Iwama et al. 2003; Grossman et al. 2007; Shoakazemi et al. 2009). These autologous bones had long-term problems including subsidence, disintegration, and infection (Shoakazemi et al. 2009; Gooch et al. 2009). Subsequently the segments of bone removed at the time of initial surgery were stored in freezers and later sterilized and replaced. Unfortunately, in a large number of patients, these plates disintegrated following their reimplantation, creating large defects. In addition to this, patients often experienced pain at the edges of the disintegrated defect. Eventually, the autologous ribs were ruled out, and various metals and acrylic-based products became increasingly used in the reconstruction (Caro-Osorio et al. 2013; Marbacher et al. 2012; Fathi et al. 2008; Shah et al. 2014). These materials required in situ molding during surgery, usually by hand or with minimal equipment. This extended the intraoperative time course and also created a number of problems including poor fit and cosmetic outcome.

When metal plates like titanium were used, these plates had to be cut and bent to fit, often ending up with sharp edges. This posed as a risk to the operating surgeon who could end up with cuts from the sharp edges. These edges and acute angling of the plates can often cause pressure on the skin flap, resulting in pain and breakdown of the overlying skin (Shah et al. 2014; Gooch et al. 2009).

3D-printed cranial implants overcome most of the problems mentioned above. Using the standard printing method described above, a mold of the decompressed segment of the skull can be created and used as the template over which a titanium plate is cut, compressed, and molded to obtain a good fit (Fig. 6.1). This individually prefabricated cranial implant is then sterilized and

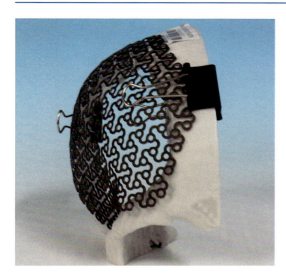

Fig. 6.1 Titanium plate compressed to 3D-printed model of defect

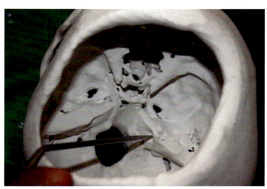

Fig. 6.2 Z Corp, Z Printer 450 printed model of the skull used to confirm spatial accuracy

implanted. In addition to titanium, other materials like acrylic and PEEK (Polyether ether ketone) have also been used to create implants using similar techniques (Caro-Osorio et al. 2013; Marbacher et al. 2012; Fathi et al. 2008; Shah et al. 2014; D'Urso et al. 2000; Rosenthal et al. 2014).

Patient's actual bone from the initial decompression cannot be used as a template at the time of implantation simply because often, the patient's skull would have undergone remodeling.

Other surgeons have also directly used 3D-printed titanium plates via the continuous deposition method. This method eliminates cutting and molding; however, these more advanced 3D printing technologies are much more expensive than earlier approaches, and the cost-benefit should be assessed among individual patient presentations (Winder et al. 1999; Dean et al. 2003).

6.4   3D-Printed Models for Surgical Simulation and Training

The first cranial models created were used to understand bone pathology as initial commercial printers like Z Corp, ZPrinter®450 (South

Carolina, USA) were only able to print in a single material that mimicked bone very well. The next step involved was in verifying the accuracy of these models both anatomically and spatially. This was performed using standard image guidance navigation stations Medtronic StealthStation®S7™System (Colorado, USA) and BrainLab Kolibri™ (Heimstetten, GER) to register 3D models of a patient's skull to the actual imaging data, thus demonstrating that surgical navigation stations were unable to distinguish the model form the actual patient. We also found all the preselected anatomical points to be spatially accurate (Waran et al. 2012) (Fig. 6.2).

As surgery on an actual patient involves not just the skeletal structures but also various soft tissue components, attempts were made to create a "face" over the facial bones that accurately reflected the patient. Initial attempts were performed using latex poured into a mold. While this technique was able to accurately create the face of a person, the process was labor intensive, and after a period of time, latex had a tendency to contract and crush the underlying "bony structures" (Fig. 6.3).

The next leap in technology was the multi-material printer. This allowed models to be printed with materials of different density like bone and soft tissue therefore creating multiple interfaces between various tissues (Stratasys Objet500 Connex™). The challenge was to enable the various tissues to interact in an "anatomical or surgical way."

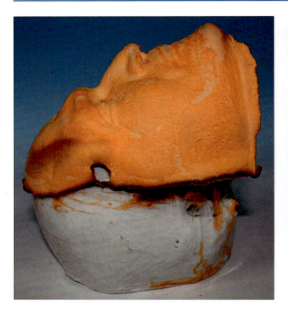

Fig. 6.3 Latex over "bone" model to mimic face

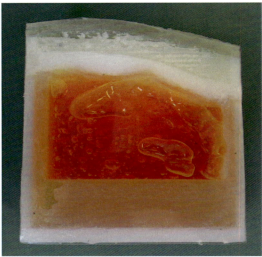

Fig. 6.4 Cross section view of the skin, skull, dura, and tumor

Multi-material printing allowed demonstration of features such as the ability to reflect skin off bone and to allow the bone to be burred or perforated using a standard craniotome, craniotome safety clutch engagement when the bone dura interface is reached and for the dura to be separated from the skull to prevent damage to underlying structures (Fig. 6.4 and Video 1).

Due to these features, we were able to successfully create models based on imaging data from actual patients with pathological findings. Our trainees are able to carry out various standard neurosurgical procedures on these models, such as:

1. Head positioning
2. Registration and planning based on neuro-navigation
3. The ability to carry out standard craniotomies including exposure and removal of simple cortical tumors (Waran et al. 2014a; Waran et al. 2014b)

The advantage of these models as surgical simulators includes the presence of original pathology within the model, as well as supporting data like proper history and medical imaging.

All standard surgical equipment used in day-to-day neurosurgery can be used, enhancing the realism of the simulator. These models provide tactile feedbacks that presently do not exist with basic box and complex virtual simulators.

Neurosurgical teaching models currently available include:

- Basic models that allow image guidance registration, flap planning, and bone flap elevation
- Stereotactic models to teach complex stereotactic planning
- Endoscopic models—both for intraventricular (Video 2) and trans-nasal surgery
- Spinal models—cervical and lumbar spine for anterior and posterior approaches (Video 3)

Despite the term multi-material, initial models worked best with one interface and two tissue densities only, for example, bone and skin.

The latest multi-material printers have allowed these models to become more dynamic. Endoscopic intraventricular models can be created with fluid-filled ventricles and intraventricular tumor. Similarly, endoscopic transsphenoidal models can be created with multiple bone ledges, intrasellar tumor, as well as cylindrical tubes cuffing the tumor to mimic carotid arteries (Figs. 6.5 and 6.6a, b).

These models have been used to run "surgical approaches workshops" and training programs for surgeons of various levels from junior trainees to senior surgeons (Narayanan et al. 2015; Waran et al. 2014b; Waran et al. 2015). With the advances in printer technology, future applications include color-printed tissues, tissues with various density, and tactile feedback that allows microdissection and cylindrical structures with pulsatile blood.

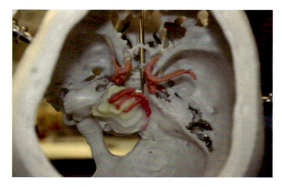

Fig. 6.5 Clival meningioma with circle of Willis

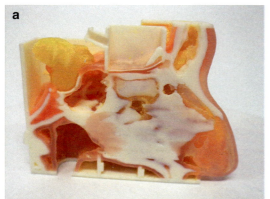

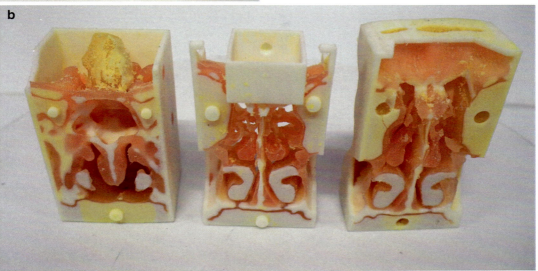

Fig. 6.6 (**a, b**) Sagittal and cross-sectional view from tip of nose to sella turcica of a patient with a pituitary tumor and an anterior water bath to mimic CSF leak

6.5 Preoperative and Intraoperative Surgical Simulation

This area has fired the imagination the most in the eyes of the public for the use of 3D printers in customized medicine. 3D printers have in the last 3–4 years been used to preoperatively plan and intraoperatively aid various complex and infrequently performed procedures. They have demonstrated their usefulness in understanding the 3D anatomy of lesions that may differ widely in appearance among individuals with similar problems.

These models have been used in the planning of pediatric neurosurgical-maxillofacial teams performing complex advancement procedures in children with cranial synostosis. Customized patient-based models are useful in the planning of individual bone cuts that are required and assess the degree of advancements that may be required (Poukens et al. 2003; Gateno et al. 2003).

Customized models have also been used in complex base of skull tumors with the aim of assessing the various surgical approaches and corridors (Kondo et al. 2016; Pacione et al. 2016; Oyama et al. 2015).

More recently, these models have been used in planning the treatment of complex vascular pathology. In this instance, the model was used to understand the complex anatomical relationship of the various vessels and related brain tissue (Ryan et al. 2016; Wurm et al. 2011; Thawani et al. 2016).

6.6 Assisting in the Consent Process

3D-printed models have shown great utility for patient consent, greatly enhancing conversations with patients and enabling meaningful explanations of pathology and interventions to patients. Surgeons have used these personally created models with in situ pathology to explain complex procedures to patients and their relatives. The surgical approaches, brain tissue within the corridor of approach, and possible complication are much better explained to a nonmedical personnel by physical models. It presents as an excellent medical aid in the consent process (Liew et al. 2015; Jones et al. 2016).

6.7 Drawbacks of 3D Printing

The main and probably only drawback of the 3D printing technology is time and cost. It requires expertise and time to segment important anatomical components individually before a print can be commenced. Printing time itself has been shortened in certain instances, but nevertheless, the 3D printing of a complex case can take up to a full day. The initial expense of buying a versatile printer and maintaining expert staff to run it is still expensive and may add on to an already escalating healthcare cost, resulting in being prohibitive to be used routinely for all patients. This current technique is therefore most useful for complex, elective procedures requiring detailed preoperative planning (Martelli et al. 2016; Ionita et al. 2014).

6.8 Conclusions

3D printing has progressed in leaps and bounds since the early days of laser-sintering resin models. We are now able to personalize models based on individual patients in an accurate and cost-effective way to help in the surgical process, surgical training, and patient understanding. The redult is that these collective technologies are very useful neurosurgical tools.

References

Caro-Osorio E, De la Garza-Ramos R, Martínez-Sánchez SR, Olazarán-Salinas F. Cranioplasty with polymethylmethacrylate prostheses fabricated by hand using original bone flaps: technical note and surgical outcomes. Surg Neurol Int. 2013;4:136.

Christensen A, Rybicki FJ. Maintaining safety and efficacy for 3D printing in medicine. 3D Print Med. 2017;3:1.

D'Urso PS, Earwaker WJ, Barker TM, Redmond MJ, Thompson RG, Effeney DJ, Tomlinson FH. Custom cranioplasty using stereolithography and acrylic. Br J Plast Surg. 2000;53(3):200–4.

Dean D, Min KJ, Bond A. Computer aided design of large-format prefabricated cranial plates. J Craniofac Surg. 2003;14(6):819–32.

Eltorai AE, Nguyen E, Daniels AH. Three-dimensional printing in orthopedic surgery. Orthopedics. 2015;38(11):684–7.

Fathi AR, Marbacher S, Lukes A. Cost-effective patient-specific intraoperative molded cranioplasty. J Craniofac Surg. 2008;19(3):777–81.

Gateno J, Teichgraeber JF, Xia JJ. Three-dimensional surgical planning for maxillary and midface distraction osteogenesis. J Craniofac Surg. 2003;14(6):833–9.

Gooch MR, Gin GE, Kenning TJ, German JW. Complications of cranioplasty following decompressive craniectomy: analysis of 62 cases. Neurosurg Focus. 2009;26(6):e9.

Grossman N, Shemesh-Jan HS, Merkin V, Gideon M, Cohen A. Deep-freeze preservation of cranial bones for future cranioplasty: nine years of experience in Soroka University Medical Center. Cell Tissue Bank. 2007;8(3):243–6.

Ionita CN, Mokin M, Varble N, Bednarek DR, Xiang J, Snyder KV, Siddiqui AH, Levy EI, Meng H, Rudin S. Challenges and limitations of patient-specific vascular phantom fabrication using 3D Polyjet printing. Proc SPIE Int Soc Opt Eng. 2014;9038:90380M.

Iwama T, Yamada J, Imai S, Shinoda J, Funakoshi T, Sakai N. The use of frozen autogenous bone flaps in delayed cranioplasty revisited. Neurosurgery. 2003;52(3):591–6. discussion 595–6.

Jones DB, Sung R, Weinberg C, Korelitz T, Andrews R. Three-dimensional modeling may improve surgical education and clinical practice. Surg Innov. 2016;23(2):189–95.

Klammert U, Gbureck U, Vorndran E, Rödiger J, Meyer-Marcotty P. Kübler AC.3D powder printed calcium phosphate implants for reconstruction of cranial and maxillofacial defects. J Craniomaxillofac Surg. 2010;38(8):565–70.

Kondo K, Harada N, Masuda H, Sugo N, Terazono S, Okonogi S, Sakaeyama Y, Fuchinoue Y, Ando S, Fukushima D, Nomoto J, Nemoto M. A neurosurgical simulation of skull base tumors using a 3D printed rapid prototyping model containing mesh structures. Acta Neurochir. 2016;158:1213.

Kozakiewicz M, Elgalal M, Loba P, Komuński P, Arkuszewski P, Broniarczyk-Loba A, Stefańczyk L. Clinical application of 3D pre-bent titanium implants for orbital floor fractures. J Craniomaxillofac Surg. 2009;37(4):229–34.

Li J, Li P, Lu H, Shen L, Tian W, Long J, Tang W. Digital design and individually fabricated titanium implants for the reconstruction of traumatic zygomatico-orbital defects. J Craniofac Surg. 2013;24(2):363–8.

Liew Y, Beveridge E, Demetriades AK, Hughes MA. 3D printing of patient-specific anatomy: a tool to improve patient consent and enhance imaging interpretation by trainees. Br J Neurosurg. 2015;29(5):712–4. doi:10.31 09/02688697.2015.1026799.

Marbacher S, Andereggen L, Erhardt S, Fathi AR, Fandino J, Raabe A, Beck J. Intraoperative template-molded bone flap reconstruction for patient-specific cranioplasty. Neurosurg Rev. 2012;35(4):527–35.

Martelli N, Serrano C, van den Brink H, Pineau J, Prognon P, Borget I, El Batti S. Advantages and disadvantages of 3-dimensional printing in surgery: a systematic review. Surgery. 2016;159:1485.

Mavili ME, Canter HI, Saglam-Aydinatay B, Kamaci S, Kocadereli I. Use of three-dimensional medical modeling methods for precise planning of orthognathic surgery. J Craniofac Surg. 2007;18(4):740–7.

McGurk M, Amis AA, Potamianos P, Goodger NM. Rapid prototyping techniques for anatomical modelling in medicine. Ann R Coll Surg Engl. 1997;79(3):169–74.

Müller A, Krishnan KG, Uhl E, Mast G. The application of rapid prototyping techniques in cranial reconstruction and preoperative planning in neurosurgery. J Craniofac Surg. 2003;14(6):899–914.

Naftulin JS, Kimchi EY, Cash SS. Streamlined, inexpensive 3D printing of the brain and skull. PLoS One. 2015;10(8):e0136198.

Narayanan V, Narayanan P, Rajagopalan R, Karuppiah R, Rahman ZA, Wormald PJ, Van Hasselt CA, Waran V. Endoscopic skull base training using 3D printed models with pre-existing pathology. Eur Arch Otorhinolaryngol. 2015;272(3):753–7.

Oyama K, Ditzel Filho LF, Muto J, de Souza DG, Gun R, Otto BA, Carrau RL, Prevedello DM. Endoscopic endonasal cranial base surgery simulation using an artificial cranial base model created by selective laser sintering. Neurosurg Rev. 2015;38(1):171–178. discussion 178. doi:10.1007/s10143-014-0580-4.

Pacione D, Tanweer O, Berman P, Harter DH. The utility of a multimaterial 3D printed model for surgical planning of complex deformity of the skull base and craniovertebral junction. J Neurosurg. 2016;125:1194.

Ploch CC, Mansi CS, Jayamohan J, Kuhl E. Using 3D printing to create personalized brain models for neurosurgical training and preoperative planning. World Neurosurg. 2016;90:668. doi:10.1016/j.wneu.2016.02.081. pii: S1878-8750(16)00326-0.

Poukens J, Haex J, Riediger D. The use of rapid prototyping in the preoperative planning of distraction osteogenesis of the cranio-maxillofacial skeleton. Comput Aided Surg. 2003;8(3):146–54.

Rengier F, Mehndiratta A, von Tengg-Kobligk H, Zechmann CM, Unterhinninghofen R, Kauczor HU, Giesel FL. 3D printing based on imaging data: review of medical applications. Int J Comput Assist Radiol Surg. 2010;5(4):335–41.

Rosenthal G, Ng I, Moscovici S, Lee KK, Lay T, Martin C, Manley GT. Polyetheretherketone implants for the repair of large cranial defects: a 3-center experience. Neurosurgery. 2014;75(5):523–9.

Rotaru H, Stan H, Florian IS, Schumacher R, Park YT, Kim SG, Chezan H, Balc N, Baciut M. Cranioplasty with custom-made implants: analyzing the cases of 10 patients. J Oral Maxillofac Surg. 2012;70(2):e169–76.

Ryan JR, Almefty K, Nakaji P, Frakes DH. Cerebral aneurysm clipping surgery simulation using patient-specific 3D printing and silicone casting. World Neurosurg. 2016;88:175. doi:10.1016/j.wneu.2015.12.102. pii: S1878-8750(16)00112-1.

Shah AM, Jung H, Skirboll S. Materials used in cranioplasty: a history and analysis. Neurosurg Focus. 2014;36(4):E19.

Shoakazemi A, Flannery T, McConnell RS. Long-term outcome of subcutaneously preserved autologous cranioplasty. Neurosurgery. 2009;65(3):505–10.

Solaro P, Pierangeli E, Pizzoni C, Boffi P, Scalese G. From computerized tomography data processing to rapid manufacturing of custom-made prostheses for cranioplasty. Case report. J Neurosurg Sci. 2008;52(4):113–6. discussion 116.

Tai BL, Rooney D, Stephenson F, Liao PS, Sagher O, Shih AJ, Savastano LE. Development of a 3D-printed external ventricular drain placement simulator: technical note. J Neurosurg. 2015;123(4):1070–6.

Thawani JP, Pisapia JM, Singh N, Petrov D, Schuster JM, Hurst RW, Zager EL, Pukenas BA. 3D-printed modeling of an arteriovenous malformation including blood flow. World Neurosurg. 2016;90:675. pii: S1878-8750(16)30022-5.

Waran V, Menon R, Pancharatnam D, Rathinam AK, Balakrishnan YK, Tung TS, Raman R, Prepageran N, Chandran H, Rahman ZA. The creation and verification of cranial models using three-dimensional rapid prototyping technology in field of transnasal sphenoid endoscopy. Am J Rhinol Allergy. 2012;26(5):e132.

Waran V, Narayanan V, Karuppiah R, Owen SL, Aziz T. Utility of multimaterial 3D printers in creating models with pathological entities to enhance the training experience of neurosurgeons. J Neurosurg. 2014a;120(2):489–92.

Waran V, Narayanan V, Karuppiah R, Pancharatnam D, Chandran H, Raman R, Rahman ZA, Owen SL, Aziz TZ. Injecting realism in surgical training-initial simulation experience with custom 3D models. J Surg Educ. 2014b;71(2):193–7.

Waran V, Narayanan V, Karuppiah R, Thambynayagam HC, Muthusamy KA, Rahman ZA, Kirollos RW. Neurosurgical endoscopic training via a realistic 3-dimensional model with pathology. Simul Healthc. 2015;10(1):43–8.

Webb PA. A review of rapid prototyping (RP) techniques in the medical and biomedical sector. J Med Eng Technol. 2000;24(4):149–53.

Winder J, Cooke RS, Gray J, Fannin T, Fegan T. Medical rapid prototyping and 3D CT in the manufacture of custom made cranial titanium plates. J Med Eng Technol. 1999;23(1):26–8.

Wurm G, Lehner M, Tomancok B, Kleiser R, Nussbaumer K. Cerebrovascular biomodeling for aneurysm surgery: simulation-based training by means of rapid prototyping technologies. Surg Innov. 2011;18(3):294–306.

Yang M, Li C, Li Y, Zhao Y, Wei X, Zhang G, Fan J, Ni H, Chen Z, Bai Y, Li M. Application of 3D rapid prototyping technology in posterior corrective surgery for Lenke 1 adolescent idiopathic scoliosis patients. Medicine (Baltimore). 2015;94(8):e582.

Zhang Z, Zhang R, Song Z. Skull defect reconstruction based on a new hybrid level set. Biomed Mater Eng. 2014;24(6):3343–51.

Zheng YX, Yu DF, Zhao JG, Wu YL, Zheng B. 3D printout models vs. 3D-rendered images: which is better for preoperative planning? J Surg Educ. 2016;73(3):518–23.

Cardiovascular 3D Printing

7

Andreas A. Giannopoulos, Dimitris Mitsouras,
Betty Anne Schwarz, Karin E. Dill,
and Frank J. Rybicki

7.1 Introduction

Cardiovascular 3D printing is now realizing its enormous potential. To date, 3D printing has been used to enhance management algorithms and plan complex cardiovascular interventions, and there is currently significant focused development for structural, valve, and congenital heart diseases, where the early evidence base supports clinical use of the technology. In the era of 3D visualization, defined as viewing various volumetric depictions on a 2D screen, spatial relationships could be assessed with new strategies but ultimately lacked the ability to convey the third dimension and tactile perception. 3D printing has extended this paradigm to a complete volumetric representation, and in cases of complex cardiovascular pathology, this "new modality" has become indispensable (Giannopoulos et al. 2016a, b; Mitsouras et al. 2015). The gamut of applications of 3D printing includes primarily planning intervention, outlined in this chapter. There are also great educational opportunities, for the radiologist, cardiologist, and surgeons, as well as patient education that will be largely addressed elsewhere in the book.

Unlike other established specialties such as orthopedics, 3D printing in the cardiovascular arena has been hampered by the paucity of 3D printing materials to simulate cardiovascular tissues. This is in stark contrast to the variety of synthetic polymers and thermoplastics that when printed resemble "hard plastics" that readily emulate bone. Nevertheless, there is significant development underway, particularly toward personalized devices and implants that are now clearly on the horizon. There is also a growing field of research enabled by 3D printing, including patient-specific flow analyses that would not be otherwise possible ex vivo. Finally, 3D printing is already established as a means to educate healthcare professionals and patients who are eager to learn more about their disease and potential interventions.

A.A. Giannopoulos (✉)
Cardiac Imaging, Department of Nuclear Medicine,
University Hospital Zurich, Raemistrasse 100,
8091 Zurich, Switzerland

Applied Imaging Science Lab, Radiology
Department, Brigham and Women's Hospital,
Harvard Medical School, Boston, MA, USA
e-mail: andgiannop@hotmail.com

D. Mitsouras
Applied Imaging Science Lab, Radiology
Department, Brigham and Women's Hospital,
Harvard Medical School, Boston, MA, USA

B.A. Schwarz • F.J. Rybicki
Department of Radiology, The University of Ottawa
Faculty of Medicine and The Ottawa Hospital
Research Institute, Ottawa, ON, Canada

K.E. Dill
Department of Radiology, University of
Massachusetts Medical School,
Worcester, MA 01655, USA

7.2   Congenital Heart Disease (CHD)

Perhaps the fastest growing applications and peer-review literature support for 3D printing are in infants with congenital heart disease. While straightforward cases of atrial (ASD) and ventricular septal defects (VSD) and patent ductus arteriosus (PDA) are routinely corrected without the benefits of 3D printing, patients with moderate and severe CHDs (6–9 per 1000 live births (Hoffman and Kaplan 2002; van der Linde et al. 2011)) will benefit from 3D printing through better surgical outcomes in terms of hemodynamics. Fluoroscopy procedures planned with 3D printed models benefit from less fluoroscopy time and lower dose of iodinated contrast use. Similarly, there is little doubt, although data collection is problematic because of lack of control data for specific procedures, that infants who have 3D printed models that can be used to plan open surgery will require less anesthesia and less time under cardiopulmonary bypass.

One key problem in CHD in general is the diverse presentation of specific pathologies; this poses challenges for surgeons and renders education very challenging. At the same time, this heterogeneity lends itself to the benefits of personalized medicine enabled by 3D printing. It is therefore not surprising that sophisticated 3D printing labs are the outgrowth of those making diagnoses and doing surgery on patients with complex CHD. Models for planning are typically printed in transparent, flexible material. This renders the ability to cut or bend the models when planning an intervention and also enables a preview of a complex surgical view that would otherwise be impossible before the procedure and entirely impossible for trainees who are scrubbed in on the case (Schrot et al. 2014) (Fig. 7.1).

The benefits of 3D printing are under-realized among the septal defects. 3D printing from CT, MRI, and 3D echocardiography, and the post-processing steps used to generate these models, is highly valuable and amendable to design patches and to navigate the direction of intraoperative occluder devices (Chaowu et al. 2016; Kim et al. 2008). 3D printing of the heart can also include

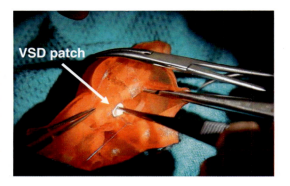

Fig. 7.1 Flexible 3D printed models of double outlet right ventricle for hands-on training of suturing the ventricular septal defect patch (photo courtesy of Prof. Shi-Joon Yoo from The Hospital for Sick Children, University of Toronto, Toronto, Canada)

the great vessels (Riesenkampff et al. 2009; Schmauss et al. 2015; Shiraishi et al. 2014, 2010; Noecker et al. 2006; Olivieri et al. 2015; Giannopoulos et al. 2015; Samuel et al. 2015). Other examples include ostium secundum ASD (Faganello et al. 2015), preoperative evaluation of ASD, and occlusion trials to avoid potentially unnecessary procedures (Chaowu et al. 2016) and VSDs (Olivieri et al. 2015). 3D printing has been used for occluder device sizing and selection of the approach to cross the defect in a congenital muscular VSD (Kim et al. 2008).

7.2.1   Complex Pediatric and Adult Congenital Heart Diseases

Reports of 3D printing benefits in congenital heart disease are now too numerous to discuss in a case-by-case format (Riesenkampff et al. 2009; Noecker et al. 2006; Matsumoto et al. 2015; Mottl-Link et al. 2008; Olivieri et al. 2014; Ryan et al. 2015; Shirakawa et al. 2016; Sodian et al. 2008; Valverde et al. 2015). The most important contribution in the field is in double outlet right ventricle (DORV) (Farooqi et al. 2016; Yoo et al. 2016a, b; Greil et al. 2007; Vodiskar et al. 2017). In addition to the variability associated with the VSD (usually present), the infundibular and intracardiac variability has resulted in individualized surgical approaches.

These have been summarized and captured in a library (IMIB-CHD n.d.) of flexible 3D printed models used to teach anatomy and the aid in several organized surgical training initiatives (Yoo et al. 2016a, b).

Tetralogy of Fallot (TOF) also has variability, and infants have greatly benefited from the availability of 3D models. Examples include TOF with pulmonary atresia, where 3D printing has been used to depict the pulmonary vascular anatomy, including collateral flow (Ryan et al. 2015) that can be referenced intraoperatively (Ngan et al. 2006). Benefits have also been realized in infants with hypoplastic left heart syndrome (Shiraishi et al. 2006, 2014; Kiraly et al. 2016) and transposition of the great vessels (Valverde et al. 2015).

7.3 Adult Heart Disease

7.3.1 Left Atrial Appendage Closure

There is an increasing need to exclude circulation within the left atrial appendage for patients with non-valvular atrial fibrillation; this can be an alternative therapy to prevent thromboembolism when there is a relative contraindication to anti-coagulation (Holmes et al. 2014). The current standard of care uses TEE with fluoroscopy guidance, and there is an increasing interest to utilize data from a pre-intervention CT, akin to other methods for atrial fibrillation therapy. The left atrial appendage has a variable anatomy, and while there are now several devices available, there can be considerable debate and uncertainty regarding the optimum device sizing. Once the decision to use a device is made clinically, sizing is of paramount importance, since there can be serious complications to a procedure that leads to incomplete occlusion or to one that uses a device whose size exceeds the tolerance of the tissue. The role of 3D printing is to assist in best-sizing the device to determine the optimum dimensions and enabling simulation and education of the procedure. The latter application will benefit from new printing materials to better emulate myocardium.

7.3.2 Hypertrophic Obstructive Cardiomyopathy

Hypertrophic obstructive cardiomyopathy has a wide spectrum of disease states but in general has the pathophysiology of eccentric and regional hypertrophy of the left ventricle (Maron et al. 2016). While most patients are treated medically, myomectomy of the ventricular septum can be performed with the intended result of reducing the obstruction to the outflow of blood to the aorta (Gersh et al. 2011; Elliott et al. 2014; Maron et al. 2011). Imaging is usually performed with cardiac MRI. 3D models offer a unique perspective of the 3D orientation of the outflow tract and key haptic anatomical feedback (Yang et al. 2015) (Fig. 7.2). In theory, a 3D model that could incorporate the systolic anterior motion from the mitral valve anterior leaflet would be highly valuable as it could be connected to a flow pump to spatially comprehend the motion and its relationship to the outflow tract throughout the cardiac cycle.

7.3.3 Cardiac Tumors

3D printing provides advanced understanding of the relationship of the unusual cardiovascular tumors for which intervention is a consideration. While 3D visualization, e.g., using customized MR acquisitions, can be adequate for delineating the myocardium, models can be useful to show the relationship between a mass and an adjacent structure that may be involved (Jacobs et al. 2008; Schmauss et al. 2013; Son et al. 2015; Al Jabbari et al. 2016).

7.3.4 Valve Disease

The last decade has seen highly innovative treatment strategies for valve disease. Two major procedures that have been enabled by technique and device advances are transcatheter aortic valve repair (TAVR) (Schmauss et al. 2012; Webb and Lauck 2016) and transcatheter mitral valve repair (TMVR). These two procedures share two main characteristics in common. First, they are far less invasive than conventional valve treatments that

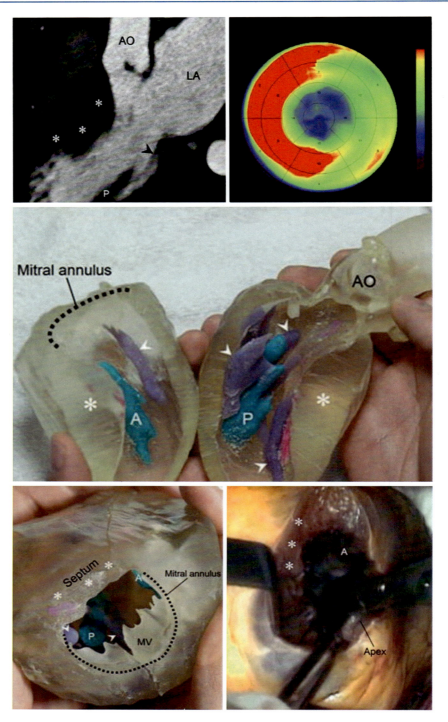

Fig. 7.2 *Top left*: Hypertrophic interventricular septum (*asterisks*), posterior papillary muscle (P), and intraventricular muscle band or accessory papillary muscles (*arrowhead*). *Top right*: Bull's eye map from end-diastolic CT demonstrating extent of hypertrophy (*red area*, >15 mm in thickness). *Middle row*: Color-coded 3D-printed model demonstrates the hypertrophic septum (*asterisks*), papillary muscle (*A* anterior, *P* posterior), and intraventricular muscle band (*asterisks*). *Bottom row*: Intraoperative view from the apical approach demonstrates the limited visual field of the LV cavity in both the model and the patient. *AO* aorta, *LA* left atrium, *LV* left ventricle, *MV* mitral valve. Yang et al. Circulation. 2015;132:300–301

use open surgery. However, the second characteristic is a consequence of the first: without surgery, there is no opportunity to visually inspect and understand the true 3D representation of the valve anatomy. This can be highly relevant as the geometry differs among patients, and the experience of the operator in these relatively new procedures is variable. Consequently, 3D printing of valve pathology has emerged as a growing field, taking advantage of the ability of 3D printing to incorporate multimodality imaging, namely, echocardiography plus CT and MRI.

The number and scope of TAVR continues to grow (Webb and Lauck 2016), and it is now established that TAVR is a generally safe alternative to surgery for many patients (Nishimura et al. 2014; Moat 2016) and has an expanding role (Webb and Lauck 2016). While some procedures are straightforward, there is mounting evidence that 3D printing has a clear role to help delineate both the anatomy and the hemodynamics of pathology, as well as the effect of calcification for patients at higher risk for complications (Gallo et al. 2016). Valvular stenosis of the aorta is already well addressed by 3D printed models, and these models can be used to plan TAVR (Maragiannis et al. 2015) (Fig. 7.3). In some patients, the procedure is

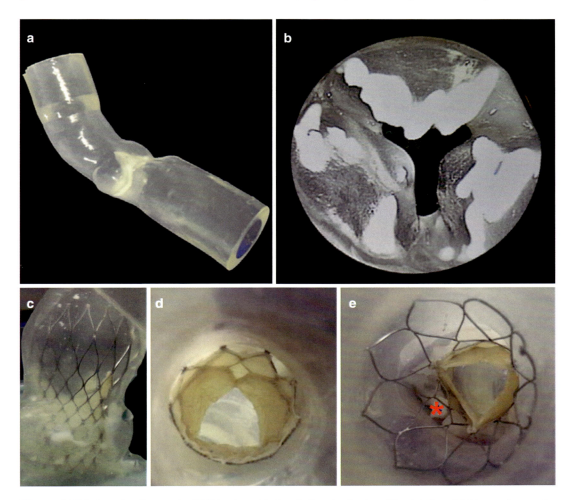

Fig. 7.3 3D Printing of aortic stenosis. 3D Printed model of a severely stenotic aortic valve derived from CT (**a, b**); aortic wall tissue is printed in flexible transparent material and calcium in opaque rigid material. Flow experiments using this model resulted in functional characteristics similar to those of in vivo assessed by spectral Doppler. Transcatheter-deployed valve in a 3D printed model (**c**) seen from endoscopic LVOT (**d**) and aortic views (**e**) demonstrate the final configuration of a self expanding stent around a calcification (*red asterisk* in **e**). Maragiannis D et al. J Am Coll Cardiol. 2014 Sep 9;64(10):1066–8 (panels **a–c**). Maragiannis D et al. Circ Cardiovasc Imaging. 2015;8:e003626 (panels **d, e**)

designed through the cardiac apex, where a printed model of the myocardium in addition to the valve can help plan intervention (Fujita et al. 2015). There is also an increasing interest in so-called "valve-in-valve procedures" where a second valve is placed within the first, generating another potential indication where a physical model can be used to classify patients into surgical versus percutaneous candidate, and when a second TAVR is considered, to determine the most accurate measurements that will lead to optimal choice of prostheses (Fujita et al. 2015).

The implementation of more flexible materials, and those that better mimic physiology in health and disease, is an important advance so that models can better emulate the impaired function of the stenosed aortic valve (Maragiannis et al. 2014). Regarding complications, there is ongoing debate regarding the significance of small paravalvular leaks. However, when a leak is characterized as moderate, there is a negative impact on valve function, as well as survival (Figulla et al. 2016). When intervention for a leak is considered the best management option, a percutaneous approach is often preferred (Sorajja et al. 2011), where models can help guide the procedure. Conversely, flexible 3D printed models of the aortic root complex derived from routine pre-TAVR CT (Dill et al. 2013) have been shown to predict paravalvular leaks after the procedure as determined by echocardiography (Ripley et al. 2016), which may help minimize this complication.

The success of less invasive interventions in the aortic valve has undoubtedly inspired approaches to treating mitral disease. Several studies support that the valve apparatus can be printed (Binder et al. 2000; Dankowski et al. 2014; Kapur and Garg 2014; Mahmood et al. 2014, 2015; Witschey et al. 2014). The imaging data required for these models is derived from echocardiography and CT, and there is growing evidence that this as an appropriate indication for 3D printing. For example, prints

of normal versus regurgitant mitral valves (Witschey et al. 2014) have been used to determine the ring selection at annuloplasty and have been used to enhance spatial understanding of the 3D relationships at surgery (Owais et al. 2014) and estimate the risk of left ventricle outflow tract obstruction (Wang et al. 2016).

Regarding transcatheter approaches, these percutaneous techniques, in theory, are lower risk than their counterpart open procedure for functional mitral regurgitation (Figulla et al. 2016). As in TAVR, though, the lower risk from avoiding an open repair comes with the cost of reduced intra-procedure visualization, and there is an unmet need to correctly size the mitral annulus and to avoid obstruction of left ventricular outflow. Literature is beginning to support models for pre-percutaneous implantation of an annuloplasty system (Dankowski et al. 2014) as well as deployment of a MitraClip (Abbott Laboratories, Abbott Park, IL) (Little et al. 2016) (Fig. 7.4).

7.4 3D Printing for the Systemic Vessels

Large vessels are readily 3D printed using flexible materials that are amendable for printing a hollow lumen with, e.g., aneurysms, mobile thrombi, and atherosclerotic plaques (Fig. 7.5); benefits span many vascular pathologies (Pepper et al. 2013; Tam et al. 2014; Itagaki 2015; Salloum et al. 2016). In addition, flow simulations using these models, printed with appropriate methods to replicate vascular compliance (Biglino et al. 2013), expand the utility of these models beyond assessing morphology alone. Common applications include aneurysms, for example, on the root of the aorta in patients with Marfan syndrome. Models enable patient-tailored approaches such as customized patch design for repair of the aorta (Izgi et al. 2015). This can minimize risk and preserve as much of the native aorta as possible (Treasure et al. 2014;

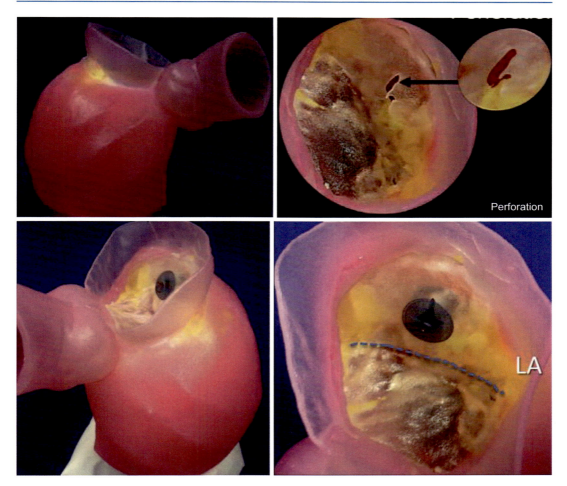

Fig. 7.4 Simulation of patient-specific mitral valve intervention using 3D printed model from CT. Model valve leaflets and the subvalvular calcium deposition (*upper left panel*) was created from CT images to assist in selection and sizing of an occluder device in a case of severe mitral valve regurgitation with restricted leaflet coaptation and a perforation of the posterior leaflet (*upper right panel*). An AMPLATZER Duct Occluder II (St. Jude Medical, St. Paul, Minnesota) was placed across the posterior leaflet perforation (*lower left panel*) and evaluated for potential interaction with the leaflet coaptation zone (*lower right panel*; superimposed dotted line). Little SH et al. JACC Cardiovasc Interv. 2016 May 9;9(9):973–5

Tam et al. 2013). Another application in the aorta is the use of 3D printing to improve outcomes in endovascular aneurysm repair, where a physical model can accurately depict complex aneurysm geometry (Tam et al. 2014; Russ et al. 2015).

Finally, 3D printing provides a uniquely strong methodology to model and test cardiovascular hemodynamics. Printed vascular models provide the opportunity for patient-specific device bench testing (Russ et al. 2015; Meess et al. 2017) and even optimization of imaging technologies and hypothesis testing that would not otherwise be possible in vivo (Mitsouras et al. 2015; Nagesh et al. 2017).

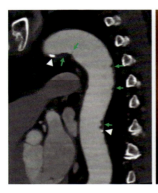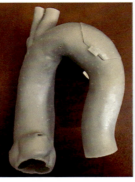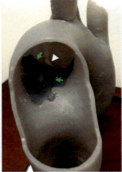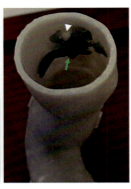

Fig. 7.5 CTA of aorta with mobile mural thrombi (*left panel*, *green arrows*) and calcifications (*left panel*, *white arrowheads*) is used to 3D-print a model that includes a cutout window that can be removed to inspect the aortic lumen to appreciate the location and size of calcifications and thrombi toward planning percutaneous intervention. Giannopoulos AA et al. J Thorac Imaging. 2016 Sep;31 (5):253–72

7.5   Conclusions

3D printing is rapidly being developed and its applications are expanding in the cardiovascular arena. Models are now routinely generated from CT and MRI images, and increasingly from 3D echocardiography. The primary use of models to date has been in surgical planning, although there is a growing interest to use models for intravascular procedure planning, outcome prediction, and even diagnosis for complicated patients. Benefits include patients with CHD, valve diseases, and in particular those amenable for newer, less invasive treatments, certain forms of structural heart disease, and for vascular pathologies particularly in the aorta. This new "modality" represents a paradigm shift from the last two decades in which 3D visualization on a 3D screen changed the way that pathology was depicted. Over the next decade to 20 years, models will be generated directly from noninvasive imaging, further simplifying management of even the most complicated patients and providing new opportunities for care pathways.

References

Al Jabbari O, Abu Saleh WK, Patel AP, Igo SR, Reardon MJ. Use of three-dimensional models to assist in the resection of malignant cardiac tumors. J Card Surg. 2016;31(9):581–3.

Biglino G, Verschueren P, Zegels R, Taylor AM, Schievano S. Rapid prototyping compliant arterial phantoms for in-vitro studies and device testing. J Cardiovasc Magn Reson. 2013;15:2.

Binder TM, Moertl D, Mundigler G, Rehak G, Franke M, Delle-Karth G, Mohl W, Baumgartner H, Maurer G. Stereolithographic biomodeling to create tangible hard copies of cardiac structures from echocardiographic data: in vitro and in vivo validation. J Am Coll Cardiol. 2000;35(1):230–7.

Chaowu Y, Hua L, Xin S. Three-dimensional printing as an aid in transcatheter closure of secundum atrial Septal defect with rim deficiency: in vitro trial occlusion based on a personalized heart model. Circulation. 2016;133(17):e608–10.

Dankowski R, Baszko A, Sutherland M, Firek L, Kalmucki P, Wroblewska K, Szyszka A, Groothuis A, Siminiak T. 3D heart model printing for preparation of percutaneous structural interventions: description of the technology and case report. Kardiol Pol. 2014;72(6):546–51.

Dill KE, George E, Abbara S, Cummings K, Francois CJ, Gerhard-Herman MD, Gornik HL, Hanley M, Kalva SP, Kirsch J, Kramer CM, Majdalany BS, Moriarty JM, Oliva IB, Schenker MP, Strax R, Rybicki FJ. ACR appropriateness criteria imaging for transcatheter aortic valve replacement. J Am Coll Radiol. 2013;10(12):957–65.

Elliott PM, Anastasakis A, Borger MA, Borggrefe M, Cecchi F, Charron P, Hagege AA, Lafont A, Limongelli G, Mahrholdt H, McKenna WJ, Mogensen J, Nihoyannopoulos P, Nistri S, Pieper PG, Pieske B, Rapezzi C, Rutten FH, Tillmanns C, Watkins H, O'Mahony C, Zamorano JL, Achenbach S, Baumgartner H, Bax JJ, Bueno H, Dean V, Deaton C, Erol Ç, Fagard R, Ferrari R, Hasdai D, Hoes AW, Kirchhof P, Knuuti J, Kolh P, Lancellotti P, Linhart A, Nihoyannopoulos P, Piepoli MF, Ponikowski P, Sirnes PA, Tamargo JL, Tendera M, Torbicki A, Wijns W, Windecker S, Hasdai D,

Ponikowski P, Achenbach S, Alfonso F, Basso C, Cardim NM, Gimeno JR, Heymans S, Holm PJ, Keren A, Kirchhof P, Kolh P, Lionis C, Muneretto C, Priori S, Salvador MJ, Wolpert C, Zamorano JL, Frick M, Aliyev F, Komissarova S, Mairesse G, Smajić E, Velchev V, Antoniades L, Linhart A, Bundgaard H, Heliö T, Leenhardt A, Katus HA, Efthymiadis G, Sepp R, Thor Gunnarsson G, Carasso S, Kerimkulova A, Kamzola G, Skouri H, Eldirsi G, Kavoliuniene A, Felice T, Michels M, Hermann Haugaa K, Lenarczyk R, Brito D, Apetrei E, Bokheria L, Lovic D, Hatala R, Garcia Pavía P, Eriksson M, Noble S, Srbinovska E, Özdemir M, Nesukay E, Sekhri N. 2014 ESC Guidelines on diagnosis and management of hypertrophic cardiomyopathy. The Task Force for the Diagnosis and Management of Hypertrophic Cardiomyopathy of the European Society of Cardiology (ESC). Eur Heart J. 2014;35(39):2733–79.

Faganello G, Campana C, Belgrano M, Russo G, Pozzi M, Cioffi G, Di Lenarda A. Three dimensional printing of an atrial septal defect: is it multimodality imaging? Int J Cardiovasc Imaging. 2015;32(3):427–8.

Farooqi KM, Uppu SC, Nguyen K, Srivastava S, Ko HH, Choueiter N, Wollstein A, Parness IA, Narula J, Sanz J, Nielsen JC. Application of virtual three-dimensional models for simultaneous visualization of intracardiac anatomic relationships in double outlet right ventricle. Pediatr Cardiol. 2016;37(1):90–8.

Figulla HR, Webb JG, Lauten A, Feldman T. The transcatheter valve technology pipeline for treatment of adult valvular heart disease. Eur Heart J. 2016;37(28):2226–39.

Fujita B, Kutting M, Scholtz S, Utzenrath M, Hakim-Meibodi K, Paluszkiewicz L, Schmitz C, Borgermann J, Gummert J, Steinseifer U, Ensminger S. Development of an algorithm to plan and simulate a new interventional procedure. Interact Cardiovasc Thorac Surg. 2015;21(1):87–95.

Gallo M, D'Onofrio A, Tarantini G, Nocerino E, Remondino F, Gerosa G. 3D-printing model for complex aortic transcatheter valve treatment. Int J Cardiol. 2016;210:139–40.

Gersh BJ, Maron BJ, Bonow RO, Dearani JA, Fifer MA, Link MS, Naidu SS, Nishimura RA, Ommen SR, Rakowski H, Seidman CE, Towbin JA, Udelson JE, Yancy CW. 2011 ACCF/AHA Guideline for the Diagnosis and Treatment of Hypertrophic Cardiomyopathy A Report of the American College of Cardiology Foundation/American Heart Association Task Force on Practice Guidelines Developed in Collaboration With the American Association for Thoracic Surgery, American Society of Echocardiography, American Society of Nuclear Cardiology, Heart Failure Society of America, Heart Rhythm Society, Society for Cardiovascular Angiography and Interventions, and Society of Thoracic Surgeons. J Am Coll Cardiol. 2011;58(25):e212–60.

Giannopoulos AA, Chepelev L, Sheikh A, Wang A, Dang W, Akyuz E, Hong C, Wake N, Pietila T, Dydynski PB, Mitsouras D, Rybicki FJ. 3D printed ventricular septal defect patch: a primer for the 2015 Radiological Society of North America (RSNA) hands-on course in 3D printing. 3D Print Med. 2015;1(1):3.

Giannopoulos AA, Mitsouras D, Yoo SJ, Liu PP, Chatzizis YS, Rybicki FJ. Applications of 3D printing in cardiovascular diseases. Nat Rev Cardiol. 2016a;13(12):701–18.

Giannopoulos AA, Steigner ML, George E, Barile M, Hunsaker AR, Rybicki FJ, Mitsouras D. Cardiothoracic applications of 3-dimensional printing. J Thorac Imaging. 2016b;31(5):253–72.

Greil GF, Wolf I, Kuettner A, Fenchel M, Miller S, Martirosian P, Schick F, Oppitz M, Meinzer HP, Sieverding L. Stereolithographic reproduction of complex cardiac morphology based on high spatial resolution imaging. Clin Res Cardiol. 2007;96(3):176–85.

Hoffman JIE, Kaplan S. The incidence of congenital heart disease. J Am Coll Cardiol. 2002;39(12):1890–900.

Holmes DR, Lakkireddy DR, Whitlock RP, Waksman R, Mack MJ. Left atrial appendage occlusion opportunities and challenges. J Am Coll Cardiol. 2014;63(4):291–8.

3DHopeMedical. IMIB-CHD. n.d.. http://imib-chd.com/.

Itagaki MW. Using 3D printed models for planning and guidance during endovascular intervention: a technical advance. Diagn Interv Radiol. 2015;21(4):338–41.

Izgi C, Nyktari E, Alpendurada F, Bruengger AS, Pepper J, Treasure T, Mohiaddin R. Effect of personalized external aortic root support on aortic root motion and distension in Marfan syndrome patients. Int J Cardiol. 2015;197:154–60.

Jacobs S, Grunert R, Mohr FW, Falk V. 3D-imaging of cardiac structures using 3D heart models for planning in heart surgery: a preliminary study. Interact Cardiovasc Thorac Surg. 2008;7(1):6–9.

Kapur KK, Garg N. Echocardiography derived three-dimensional printing of normal and abnormal mitral annuli. Ann Card Anaesth. 2014;17(4):283–4.

Kim MS, Hansgen AR, Wink O, Quaife RA, Carroll JD. Rapid prototyping: a new tool in understanding and treating structural heart disease. Circulation. 2008;117(18):2388–94.

Kiraly L, Tofeig M, Jha NK, Talo H. Three-dimensional printed prototypes refine the anatomy of post-modified Norwood-1 complex aortic arch obstruction and allow presurgical simulation of the repair. Interact Cardiovasc Thorac Surg. 2016;22(2):238–40.

van der Linde D, Konings EE, Slager MA, Witsenburg M, Helbing WA, Takkenberg JJ, Roos-Hesselink JW. Birth prevalence of congenital heart disease worldwide: a systematic review and meta-analysis. J Am Coll Cardiol. 2011;58(21):2241–7.

Little SH, Vukicevic M, Avenatti E, Ramchandani M, Barker CM. 3D printed modeling for patient-specific mitral valve intervention: repair with a clip and a plug. JACC Cardiovasc Interv. 2016;9(9):973–5.

Mahmood F, Owais K, Montealegre-Gallegos M, Matyal R, Panzica P, Maslow A, Khabbaz KR. Echocardiography derived three-dimensional printing of normal and abnormal mitral annuli. Ann Card Anaesth. 2014;17(4):279–83.

Mahmood F, Owais K, Taylor C, Montealegre-Gallegos M, Manning W, Matyal R, Khabbaz KR. Three-dimensional printing of mitral valve using echocardiographic data. JACC Cardiovasc Imaging. 2015;8(2):227–9.

Maragiannis D, Jackson MS, Igo SR, Chang SM, Zoghbi WA, Little SH. Functional 3D printed patient-specific modeling of severe aortic stenosis. J Am Coll Cardiol. 2014;64(10):1066–8.

Maragiannis D, Jackson MS, Igo SR, Schutt RC, Connell P, Grande-Allen J, Barker CM, Chang SM, Reardon MJ, Zoghbi WA, Little SH. Replicating patient-specific severe aortic valve stenosis with functional 3D modeling. Circ Cardiovasc Imaging. 2015;8(10):e003626.

Maron BJ, Yacoub M, Dearani JA. Benefits of surgery in obstructive hypertrophic cardiomyopathy: bring septal myectomy back for European patients. Eur Heart J. 2011;32(9):1055–8.

Maron BJ, Rowin EJ, Casey SA, Maron MS. How hypertrophic cardiomyopathy became a contemporary treatable genetic disease with low mortality: shaped by 50 years of clinical research and practice. JAMA Cardiol. 2016;1(1):98–105.

Matsumoto JS, Morris JM, Foley TA, Williamson EE, Leng S, McGee KP, Kuhlmann JL, Nesberg LE, Vrtiska TJ. Three-dimensional physical modeling: applications and experience at Mayo Clinic. Radiographics. 2015;35(7):1989–2006.

Meess KM, Izzo RL, Dryjski ML, Curl RE, Harris LM, Springer M, Siddiqui AH, Rudin S, Ionita CN. 3D printed abdominal aortic aneurysm phantom for image guided surgical planning with a patient specific fenestrated endovascular graft system. In: Proc. SPIE 10138, medical imaging 2017: imaging informatics for healthcare, research, and applications, Orlando, FL, 2017.

Mitsouras D, Liacouras P, Imanzadeh A, Giannopoulos AA, Cai T, Kumamaru KK, George E, Wake N, Caterson EJ, Pomahac B, Ho VB, Grant GT, Rybicki FJ. Medical 3D printing for the radiologist. Radiographics. 2015;35(7):1965–88.

Moat NE. Will TAVR become the predominant method for treating severe aortic stenosis? N Engl J Med. 2016;374(17):1682–3.

Mottl-Link S, Hubler M, Kuhne T, Rietdorf U, Krueger JJ, Schnackenburg B, De Simone R, Berger F, Juraszek A, Meinzer HP, Karck M, Hetzer R, Wolf I. Physical models aiding in complex congenital heart surgery. Ann Thorac Surg. 2008;86(1):273–7.

Nagesh SV, Russ M, Ionita CN, Bednarek D, Rudin S. Use of patient specific 3D printed neurovascular phantoms to evaluate the clinical utility of a high resolution X-ray imager. In: Proc SPIE Int Soc Opt Eng, vol 10137: biomedical applications in molecular, structural, and functional imaging, Orlando, FL, 2017.

Ngan EM, Rebeyka IM, Ross DB, Hirji M, Wolfaardt JF, Seelaus R, Grosvenor A, Noga ML. The rapid prototyping of anatomic models in pulmonary atresia. J Thorac Cardiovasc Surg. 2006;132(2):264–9.

Nishimura RA, Otto CM, Bonow RO, Carabello BA, Erwin IIIJP, Guyton RA, O'Gara PT, Ruiz CE, Skubas NJ, Sorajja P, Sundt IIITM, Thomas JD. 2014 AHA/ACC guideline for the management of patients with valvular heart disease: a report of the American College of Cardiology/American Heart Association Task Force on Practice Guidelines. J Am Coll Cardiol. 2014;63(22):e57–e185.

Noecker AM, Chen JF, Zhou Q, White RD, Kopcak MW, Arruda MJ, Duncan BW. Development of patient-specific three-dimensional pediatric cardiac models. ASAIO J. 2006;52(3):349–53.

Olivieri L, Krieger A, Chen MY, Kim P, Kanter JP. 3D heart model guides complex stent angioplasty of pulmonary venous baffle obstruction in a Mustard repair of D-TGA. Int J Cardiol. 2014;172(2):e297–8.

Olivieri LJ, Krieger A, Loke YH, Nath DS, Kim PC, Sable CA. Three-dimensional printing of intracardiac defects from three-dimensional echocardiographic images: feasibility and relative accuracy. J Am Soc Echocardiogr. 2015;28(4):392–7.

Owais K, Pal A, Matyal R, Montealegre-Gallegos M, Khabbaz KR, Maslow A, Panzica P, Mahmood F. Three-dimensional printing of the mitral annulus using echocardiographic data: science fiction or in the operating room next door? J Cardiothorac Vasc Anesth. 2014;28(5):1393–6.

Pepper J, Petrou M, Rega F, Rosendahl U, Golesworthy T, Treasure T. Implantation of an individually computer-designed and manufactured external support for the Marfan aortic root. Multimed Man Cardiothorac Surg. 2013;2013:mmt004.

Riesenkampff E, Rietdorf U, Wolf I, Schnackenburg B, Ewert P, Huebler M, Alexi-Meskishvili V, Anderson RH, Engel N, Meinzer HP, Hetzer R, Berger F, Kuehne T. The practical clinical value of three-dimensional models of complex congenitally malformed hearts. J Thorac Cardiovasc Surg. 2009;138(3):571–80.

Ripley B, Kelil T, Cheezum MK, Goncalves A, Di Carli MF, Rybicki FJ, Steigner M, Mitsouras D, Blankstein R. 3D printing based on cardiac CT assists anatomic visualization prior to transcatheter aortic valve replacement. J Cardiovasc Comput Tomogr. 2016;10(1):28–36.

Russ M, O'Hara R, Setlur Nagesh SV, Moki M, Jimenez C, Siddiqui A, Bednarek D, Rudin S, Ionita C. Treatment planning for image-guided neuro-vascular interventions using patient-specific 3D printed phantoms. Proc SPIE Int Soc Opt Eng. 2015;9417:941726.

Ryan JR, Moe TG, Richardson R, Frakes DH, Nigro JJ, Pophal S. A novel approach to neonatal management of tetralogy of Fallot, with pulmonary atresia, and multiple aortopulmonary collaterals. JACC Cardiovasc Imaging. 2015;8(1):103–4.

Salloum C, Lim C, Fuentes L, Osseis M, Luciani A, Azoulay D. Fusion of information from 3D printing and surgical robot: an innovative minimally technique illustrated by the resection of a large celiac trunk aneurysm. World J Surg. 2016;40(1):245–7.

Samuel BP, Pinto C, Pietila T, Vettukattil JJ. Ultrasound-derived three-dimensional printing in congenital heart disease. J Digit Imaging. 2015;28(4):459–61.

Schmauss D, Schmitz C, Bigdeli AK, Weber S, Gerber N, Beiras-Fernandez A, Schwarz F, Becker C, Kupatt C, Sodian R. Three-dimensional printing of models for preoperative planning and simulation of transcatheter valve replacement. Ann Thorac Surg. 2012;93(2):e31–3.

Schmauss D, Gerber N, Sodian R. Three-dimensional printing of models for surgical planning in patients with primary cardiac tumors. J Thorac Cardiovasc Surg. 2013;145(5):1407–8.

Schmauss D, Haeberle S, Hagl C, Sodian R. Three-dimensional printing in cardiac surgery and interventional cardiology: a single-centre experience. Eur J Cardiothorac Surg. 2015;47(6):1044–52.

Schrot J, Pietila T, Sahu A. State of the art: 3D printing for creating compliant patient-specific congenital heart defect models. J Cardiovasc Magn Reson. 2014;16(Suppl 1):W19.

Shiraishi I, Kajiyama Y, Yamagishi M, Hamaoka K. Images in cardiovascular medicine. Stereolithographic biomodeling of congenital heart disease by multislice computed tomography imaging. Circulation. 2006;113(17):e733–4.

Shiraishi I, Yamagishi M, Hamaoka K, Fukuzawa M, Yagihara T. Simulative operation on congenital heart disease using rubber-like urethane stereolithographic biomodels based on 3D datasets of multislice computed tomography. Eur J Cardiothorac Surg. 2010;37(2):302–6.

Shiraishi I, Kurosaki K, Kanzaki S, Ichikawa H. Development of super flexible replica of congenital heart disease with stereolithography 3D printing for simulation surgery and medical education. J Card Fail. 2014;20(10):S180–1.

Shirakawa T, Koyama Y, Mizoguchi H, Yoshitatsu M. Morphological analysis and preoperative simulation of a double-chambered right ventricle using 3-dimensional printing technology. Interact Cardiovasc Thorac Surg. 2016;22(5):688–90.

Sodian R, Weber S, Markert M, Loeff M, Lueth T, Weis FC, Daebritz S, Malec E, Schmitz C, Reichart B. Pediatric cardiac transplantation: three-dimensional printing of anatomic models for surgical planning of heart transplantation in patients with univentricular heart. J Thorac Cardiovasc Surg. 2008;136(4):1098–9.

Son KH, Kim KW, Ahn CB, Choi CH, Park KY, Park CH, Lee JI, Jeon YB. Surgical planning by 3D printing for primary cardiac schwannoma resection. Yonsei Med J. 2015;56(6):1735–7.

Sorajja P, Cabalka AK, Hagler DJ, Rihal CS. Long-term follow-up of percutaneous repair of paravalvular prosthetic regurgitation. J Am Coll Cardiol. 2011;58(21):2218–24.

Tam MD, Laycock SD, Brown JR, Jakeways M. 3D printing of an aortic aneurysm to facilitate decision making and device selection for endovascular aneurysm repair in complex neck anatomy. J Endovasc Ther. 2013;20(6):863–7.

Tam MD, Latham T, Brown JR, Jakeways M. Use of a 3D printed hollow aortic model to assist EVAR planning in a case with complex neck anatomy: potential of 3D printing to improve patient outcome. J Endovasc Ther. 2014;21(5):760–2.

Treasure T, Takkenberg JJ, Golesworthy T, Rega F, Petrou M, Rosendahl U, Mohiaddin R, Rubens M, Thornton W, Lees B, Pepper J. Personalised external aortic root support (PEARS) in Marfan syndrome: analysis of 1-9 year outcomes by intention-to-treat in a cohort of the first 30 consecutive patients to receive a novel tissue and valve-conserving procedure, compared with the published results of aortic root replacement. Heart. 2014;100(12):969–75.

Valverde I, Gomez G, Gonzalez A, Suarez-Mejias C, Adsuar A, Coserria JF, Uribe S, Gomez-Cia T, Hosseinpour AR. Three-dimensional patient-specific cardiac model for surgical planning in Nikaidoh procedure. Cardiol Young. 2015;25(4):698–704.

Vodiskar J, Kutting M, Steinseifer U, Vazquez-Jimenez JF, Sonntag SJ. Using 3D physical modeling to plan surgical corrections of complex congenital heart defects. Thorac Cardiovasc Surg. 2017;65(1):31–5.

Wang DD, Eng M, Greenbaum A, Myers E, Forbes M, Pantelic M, Song T, Nelson C, Divine G, Taylor A, Wyman J, Guerrero M, Lederman RJ, Paone G, O'Neill W. Predicting LVOT obstruction after TMVR. JACC Cardiovasc Imaging. 2016;9(11):1349–52.

Webb JG, Lauck S. Transcatheter aortic valve replacement in transition. JACC Cardiovasc Interv. 2016;9(11):1159–60.

Witschey WR, Pouch AM, McGarvey JR, Ikeuchi K, Contijoch F, Levack MM, Yushkevick PA, Sehgal CM, Jackson BM, Gorman RC, Gorman JH 3rd. Three-dimensional ultrasound-derived physical mitral valve modeling. Ann Thorac Surg. 2014;98(2):691–4.

Yang DH, Kang JW, Kim N, Song JK, Lee JW, Lim TH. Myocardial 3-dimensional printing for septal myectomy guidance in a patient with obstructive hypertrophic cardiomyopathy. Circulation. 2015;132(4):300–1.

Yoo S, Thabit O, Kim E, Ide H, Dragulescu A, Seed M, Grosse-Wortmann L, van Arsdell G. 3D printing in medicine of congenital heart diseases. 3D Print Med. 2016a;2:2.

Yoo S-J, Thabit O, Kim EK, Ide H, Yim D, Dragulescu A, Seed M, Grosse-Wortmann L, van Arsdell G. 3D printing in medicine of congenital heart diseases. 3D Print Med. 2016b;2(1):1–12.

Musculoskeletal 3D Printing

8

Satheesh Krishna, Kirstin Small, Troy Maetani, Leonid Chepelev, Betty Anne Schwarz, and Adnan Sheikh

The optimal management of musculoskeletal disease is dependent on the preservation of anatomic structures and maintenance of biomechanical and kinetic function. 3D printing is being used for presurgical planning of bone lesion resection, joint repair and replacement, congenital deformity correction, and posttraumatic fixation. It has also been utilized for therapeutic purposes through creation of patient personalized prosthetics, drug delivery systems, fixation devices, and other musculoskeletal implants.

3D printing has greatly impacted orthopedic and spine surgery; a recent systematic review shows that 53% of all published manuscripts in the last 15 years has been from the domains of orthopedics and spine surgery (Tack et al. 2016). Orthopedic models can be printed from both CT and MR images as well as from fused image sets; for example, a diagnostic

S. Krishna (✉) • L. Chepelev
Department of Medical Imaging, The Ottawa Hospital, University of Ottawa, Ottawa, ON, Canada
e-mail: sjeyaraj@toh.ca

K. Small, M.D.
Department of Radiology, Brigham and Women's Hospital and Harvard Medical School,
Boston, MA, USA

T. Maetani, M.D.
Department of Radiology, UNC School of Medicine, Chapel Hill, NC, USA

B.A. Schwarz • A. Sheikh
Department of Medical Imaging, The University of Ottawa Faculty of Medicine and The Ottawa Hospital Research Institute, Ottawa, ON, Canada

MRI fused with CT images acquired for biopsy guidance. It is also possible to co-register T2-weighted sequences over post-contrast sequences over an MR angiogram to segment out the cystic/necrotic component, enhancing component and vascular structures, respectively. The applications of 3D printing in orthopedics have rapidly progressed in the last few years. This chapter highlights orthopedic applications of 3D printing.

3D printing effectively addresses many current educational shortcomings and enhances traditional methods of teaching human anatomy. 3D printed models are durable, easy to reproduce, and cost-effective. They help to avoid health and safety issues associated with wet fixed cadaver specimens (McMenamin et al. 2014). 3D models avoid problems with availability of cadaveric specimens. This is especially important for teaching anatomic variants, congenital malformations, or pathological specimens as an image set generated from one patient can be shared via online repositories and can be locally printed. This technology has been used with great success in the education of acetabular fractures (Manganaro et al. 2017). A recent randomized control trial conclusively proved that students taught anatomy by use of inexpensive 3D printed skull models scored significantly higher compared with students taught using cadaveric skulls and an anatomic atlas (Chen et al. 2017). Cadaveric specimens are limited in the study of biomechanics, while portable 3D patient-specific models can be custom generated

© Springer International Publishing AG 2017
F.J. Rybicki, G.T. Grant (eds.), *3D Printing in Medicine*, DOI 10.1007/978-3-319-61924-8_8

with movable parts replicating normal anatomy and hence are excellent complementary tools to study biomechanics. In addition to medical student education, 3D models can be an important tool in facilitating informed consent between physicians and patients, educating patients regarding their pathology, and providing an easily comprehensible visualization of treatment options including complex interventions (Bizzotto et al. 2016a, b).

In addition to providing three-dimensional visual stimulus, a 3D printed model also provides crucial tactile stimulus. This can be exploited to great advantage, especially in the field of surgery where patient-specific 3D printed models allow for surgical rehearsal. Depending on the material used for fabrication, the model can be generated to have properties similar to the corresponding anatomical tissue including firmness, texture, and elasticity. Such models can afford the opportunity to safely practice and refine surgical skills during surgical residency, greatly improving confidence and precision when subsequently actually operating on a patient. Such models also help test surgical decision-making through patient-case 3D models, and allows direct evaluation of procedural skills by an experienced attending surgeon. As the number of models are restricted only by the capacity of the 3D printer, all trainees can get enough cutting exposure, and surgical techniques can be practiced repetitively. Even experienced surgeons can benefit from models to familiarize themselves with newer surgical instruments and newer implantation hardware prior to entering the operating room.

Phantoms can also be 3D printed for specific procedural training, such as to practice lumbar spine injections or ultrasound-guided biopsy procedures. It is also possible to print 3D models of spines with scoliosis, ankylosing spondylitis, or extensive degenerative diseases. In these patients, a spinal injection my potentially be challenging (Fig. 8.1). 3D models of this type have the potential to serve as important training tools in a wide spectrum of

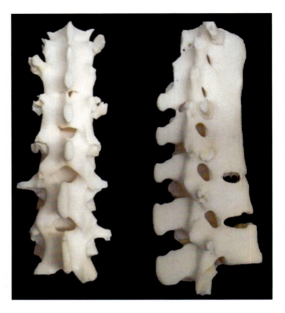

Fig. 8.1 3D model of the spine of a patient with ankylosing spondylitis showing ossification of the anterior and posterior longitudinal ligaments and ligamentum flavum. This can be used for teaching and practicing spinal interventions

regional anesthesia, guided interventions and interventional therapies, and pain management procedures (West et al. 2014).

3D printing has been increasingly used to preoperatively characterize complex anatomy. Realistic models aid in understanding complex spatial relationships resulting in accurate presurgical planning as precise preoperative measurements are obtained (Fig. 8.2). Thereby, intraoperative time can be significantly reduced. Reduced intraoperative time leads to better utilization of resources and is advantageous as longer operative times have been linked to worse outcomes. Simulated rehearsal of complex surgical steps on 3D models may decrease intraoperative complications. Fixation hardware can be positioned over the patient's 3D model and pre-contoured to ensure an optimal intraoperative fit. Current applications of 3D printing in presurgical planning include presurgical planning for lesion resection, joint repair and replacement, surgical correction of congenital musculoskeletal deformities, and surgical

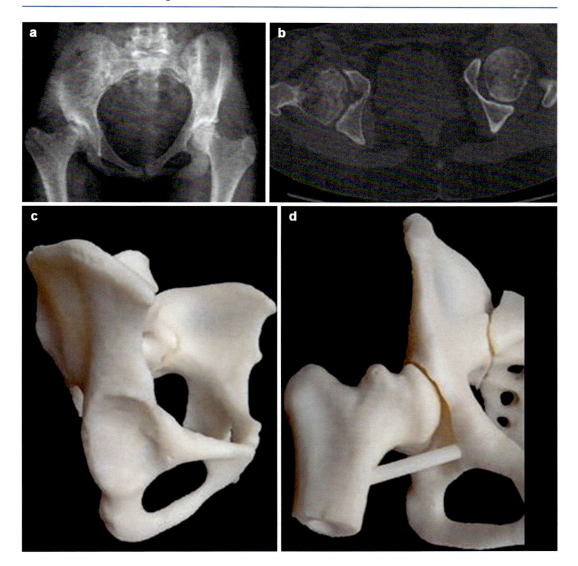

Fig. 8.2 20-year-old female with acetabular dysplasia. (**a**) Radiograph and (**b**) CT demonstrate shallow acetabulum with uncovering of the femoral heads. (**c**, **d**) 3D model provides a much greater impression of the femoral head and acetabular surface

management of osseous trauma, and are discussed as follows.

3D printing has proven beneficial in resection of large osteochondroma of the scapula where determining the precise relationship between the mass and the serratus anterior helped avoid potential postoperative scapular wing complication (Tam et al. 2012). In a more complex case, 3D printing was used to successfully carry out en bloc resection of cervical spine primary bone tumors (Xiao et al. 2016). Other degrees of complexity have been described (Kang et al. 2015; Wong et al. 2007a, b; Ma et al. 2016). Utilizing surface characteristics and spatial adjacency of landmarks, 3D bone models reconstructed from CT images have been used to localize and identify critical patient-specific anatomic landmarks (Subburaj et al. 2009). This adds invaluable anatomic information in preoperative planning when identifying important adjacent structures to avoid, such as nerves and vessels.

The intraosseous extent of tumor infiltration needs to be accurately evaluated preoperatively to ensure adequate clearance margin while minimizing the amount of resected bone (Fig. 8.3). This is of paramount importance in patients in whom joint sparing resections are planned. 3D modeling has been used in craniofacial fibrous dysplasia to direct the extent of bone shaving resection while optimizing cosmetic symmetric facial contouring with accurate surgical reduction

and shortening of operative time with the use of 3D models (Kang et al. 2015).

Functionally successful surgeries involving extremity and pelvic resections are dependent on utilizing custom prostheses to provide near anatomic restoration of function. After obtaining adequate oncologic clearance, further resection needs to be fashioned, so as to snugly accommodate the prosthesis (Wong et al. 2007a, b). An accurate fit of a custom prosthesis depends on precise measurements obtained during presurgical planning so that an apt patient-specific

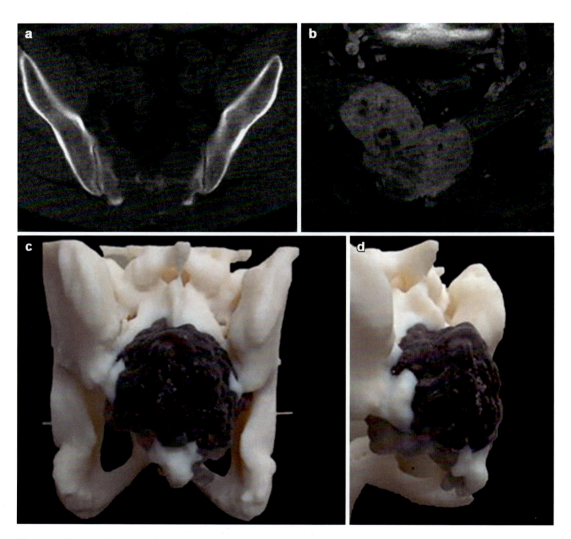

Fig. 8.3 40-year-old man with sacral chordoma. (**a**) CT and (**b**) MRI of the pelvis show a large sacral mass with sacral destruction. (**c**, **d**) 3D model better delineates the margins and extent of osseous involvement which is crucial for presurgical planning and helps in patient education

customized prosthesis can be designed. In such patients, two 3D models may need to be printed, one to plan for tumor resection and the other to help guide custom prosthesis planning (Kang et al. 2015).

3D models can be used to select optimum operative hardware, for example, in selection of optimal fixation screw based on a predetermined entry point and expected drill vector during pelvic surgery (Peters et al. 2002). 3D modeling can help design patient-specific instruments (PSI) for intraoperative guidance. Such PSI simplify complex surgical procedures, help making smaller incision size, improve precision of resection, and decrease intraoperative blood loss and overall operating time (Wong et al. 2007a, b). Designing of PSI requires postprocessing extrapolations based on dimensional and geometric specifications which can be further pre-fitted on the preoperative 3D models for further refinement to perfectly align with patient anatomy. They are subsequently used intraoperatively to deliver bone cuts in the target planes resulting in improved accuracy during complex resections (Figs. 8.4 and 8.5). PSI are especially important in pelvic resections where there is limited working space, complex geometry, and decreased intraoperative visibility (Cartiaux et al. 2014).

PSI have been used in resection of pediatric proximal tibial sarcomas (Bellanova et al. 2013), chondrosarcoma of the superior pubic ramus (Blakeney et al. 2014), and distal femoral osteosarcoma (Ma et al. 2016) among many others.

There is an increasing demand to optimize patient-specific hardware of total joint arthroplasty. It is expected that best quality of life can be achieved by personalized medicine, by fashioning hardware specific to a patient, as against a commercially mass-manufactured prosthesis, due to minor anatomic variations between patients. Patient-specific MRI or CT data define the mechanical and anatomic axes across the joint in planning for an arthroplasty. This data is used to generate the 3D model to accurately plan the size and position of the implant and to fashion a custom implant. In the arena of total joint replacements, 3D printing has led to fashioning custom total joints, intraoperative computer-assisted navigation and surgical guide systems, and PSI which encompasses pinning guides and cutting jigs (Jun 2010; Krishnan et al. 2012). In total knee arthroplasty, tibial and femoral models help create patient-specific cutting guides for preparation of the bone. These custom-made jigs attach to the underlying bone and have slits in their structure which allow cutting through them.

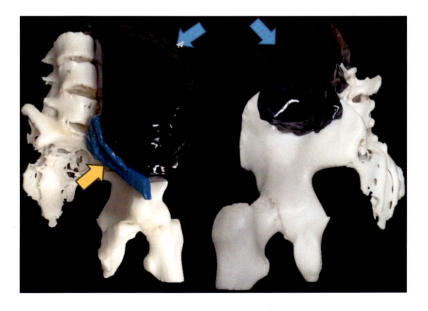

Fig. 8.4 Large soft tissue sarcoma (*blue arrows*) with iliac bone destruction. 3D model better shows bone involvement and relationship to iliac vessels (*yellow arrow*) for presurgical planning

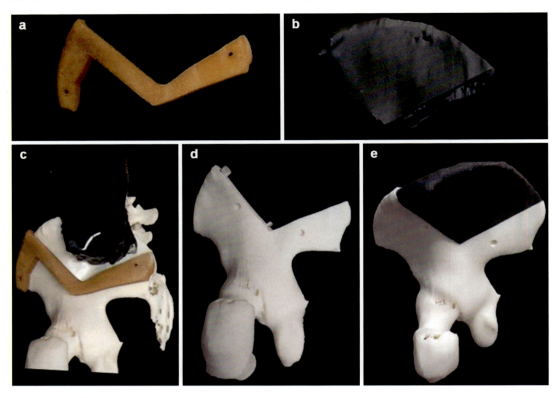

Fig. 8.5 (**a**) Patient-specific cutting guide and (**b**) iliac prosthesis for pelvic reconstruction in the same patient from Fig. 8.4, designed using mirroring techniques. (**c**) The autoclavable guide printed using ULTEM can be placed intraoperatively for precise surgical incision. (**d**) 3D models show pelvis after resection. (**e**) Hemipelvis after implant placement

Pinning guides help guide accurate pin placement to secure the jigs (Fig. 8.6).

3D models are especially useful in complex cases of arthroplasty where significant degenerative changes or large areas of bone loss result in complex anatomy. Such altered anatomy requires significant presurgical planning to determine resection level and angle of resection to ensure adequate postsurgical alignment (Schwartz et al. 2015). Minns et al. report positive surgical outcome with the help of 3D models in a patient with rheumatoid arthritis and status post Benjamin's double osteotomy that had resulted in an unstable varus deformity of the knee and marked deformity of the medial tibial plateau (Minns et al. 2003). 3D models help to predict feasibility, establish optimal surgical strategy, and select the appropriate implant type, size, and position in technically challenging total hip replacements in patients with severe acetabular deficiencies that require structural bone grafting and custom prosthetics and in cases of ankylosis (Won et al. 2013).

Revision total joint arthroplasties are technically challenging due to altered anatomy, decreased available bone stock, and difficulty in achieving stable fixation (Makinen et al. 2016). 3D models aid in presurgical planning of these complex surgeries and assist in the selection of optimum hardware or creation of patient-specific hardware (Fig. 8.7). Cage reconstruction has been utilized to gain rigid fixation in the host bone and bone graft in revision hip arthroplasties. 3D models define the available bone stock, pre-fit the cage construct, and guide surgical technique which decrease the risk of mechanical failure following revision surgery (Li et al. 2013).

Fig. 8.6 Patient-specific femoral cutting guide for optimal positioning for knee arthroplasty

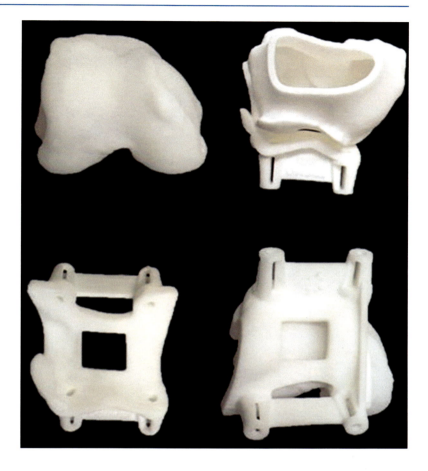

This technology has been applied to other joints such as rheumatoid arthritis cervical spine fixation and Charcot neuroarthropathy with encouraging results. Cervical spine fixation in rheumatoid arthritis is challenging due to severe deformity, erosive changes, poor bone quality, and aberrant vertebral vasculature. Full-scale 3D models of the cervical spine provide patient-specific stereoscopic mapping of complex anatomy allowing for preoperative fitting of the plate-rod construct for occipitocervical fixation. This optimizes patient alignment and defines parameters for pedicle screw trajectory and point of entry prior to surgery. Such detailed preoperative planning has been shown to decrease postoperative complications such as dysphagia (Mizutani et al. 2008). In Charcot arthropathy, 3D models allow rehearsal of incision site selection, selection of most appropriate instrumentation, determination of feasibility of

osteotomy and joint resection levels, and pre-fitting and placement of internal and external fixation devices (Giovinco et al. 2012).

Fabrication of 3D models can allow assessment of joint biomechanics prior to repair. 3D printing can be utilized to quantify the bone loss of the osseous Bankart and Hill-Sachs lesion in a patient with recurrent anterior shoulder instability. Further, 3D model helps determine the degree of abduction and external rotation at which the Hill-Sachs lesion engages. This helps guide appropriate surgical treatment, including the number of suture anchors required for the remplissage procedure and the number of anchors that would fit within the Hill-Sachs (Sheth et al. 2015).

Surgical correction of severe scoliosis is challenging due to loss of traditional anatomic landmarks, risk of major neurologic damage, risk of vascular injury, and unexpected malformations

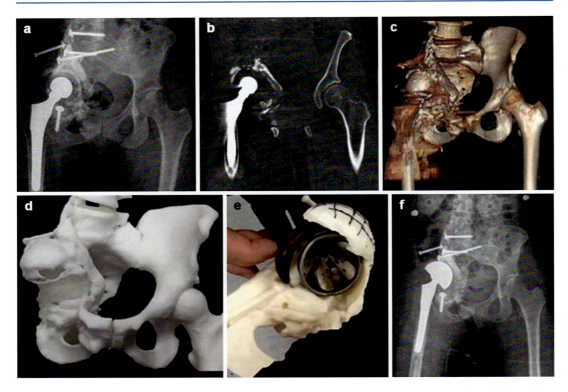

Fig. 8.7 50-year-old female with prior pelvic resection and right hip reconstruction. (**a**) Radiograph, (**b**) CT coronal image, and (**c**) CT volume rendering show displacement of the acetabular cup and hardware loosening with associated fractures of the posterior column and the inferior pubic ramus. (**d**) 3D printed model helped to better analyze the complex spatial orientation of the various components for optimal revision surgery. (**e**) The model also helped selection of optimal hardware prior to the procedure. This resulted in significant reduction in intraoperative time. (**f**) Postoperative radiograph shows revised hip arthroplasty with acetabular reconstruction

that are often only discovered during surgery, subsequently resulting in prolonged operative time, higher rate of screw misplacement, and increased risk of additional complications. In patients with congenital scoliosis, 3D computed reconstructions have been shown to be more helpful than plain radiographs in identifying posterior vertebral anomalies associated with hemivertebrae (Hedequist and Emans 2003). 3D printing can be more beneficial than 3D computed reconstructions as they allow for comprehensive presurgical evaluation and eliminate risk of encountering unexpected malformations intraoperatively. Further, they provide tactile feedback that can be used in direct rehearsal to refine surgical approach (Mao et al. 2010). The use of 3D printing technology with intraoperative fluoroscopy reduces the risk of transpedicular screw

misplacement in patients with scoliosis and its subsequent complications (Wu et al. 2011). These basic principles can be beneficially applied to other congenital pediatric musculoskeletal disorders such as pediatric hip deformities, Blount's disease, posttraumatic physeal bars, and subtalar coalitions (Starosolski et al. 2013).

3D models have proven important for complex fracture management, improved fracture characterization, more precise anatomic measurements, reduced surgical time (related to precontoured fixation hardware, 3D printed patient-specific surgical template guides, preplanned trajectory, pre-planned type and length of fixation screws), decreased anesthetic dosage requirement, and reduction in intraoperative blood loss and fluoroscopy time (Bagaria et al. 2011; Bizzotto et al. 2015; Wu et al. 2015; Brown et al. 2003). Examples include distal radial fractures, where 3D models provide better appreciation of articular surface gaps ≥2 mm and enable preoperative selection of appropriate fixation hardware (Bizzotto et al. 2016a, b). Similarly in radial head fractures, 3D models increase sensitivity in the diagnosis of fracture line separation of the head from the radial neck, radial neck comminution, articular surface involvement, articular fracture gap greater than 2 mm step-off, impacted fracture fragments, presence of greater than three articular fragments, and presence of articular fracture fragments too small to repair (Guitton et al. 2014). This results in improved consensus in fracture classification and decreased variability in surgical treatment. In chronic fracture deformities like cubitus varus, 3D models help in precise preoperative measurements for the proper location of the osteotomy, amount of wedging required, and the tilting plane of the osteotomy cut, leading to positive results in the restoration of anatomic alignment, functional postoperative outcome, and cosmetic appearance (Mahaisavariya et al. 2006).

Classification and surgical management of complex pelvic and acetabular fractures based on two-dimensional CT images is notoriously difficult. 3D models decrease the degree of interobserver variability in fracture classification and

allow for customization of proposed fixation hardware (Hurson et al. 2007; Zeng et al. 2016). For example, in type C pelvic fractures, use of 3D models decreased length of hospital stay and morbidity and accelerated recovery (Li et al. 2015). Pre-contouring of the fracture fixation plates on the mirrored healthy pelvis eliminates the need for intraoperative contouring while treating both-column acetabular fractures, thereby reducing intraoperative time (Upex et al. 2017). 3D printed pelvic osseous models can be overlaid with vascular information obtained from CT angiography. Printed pelvic arteries and veins can be layered in anatomic relation to the fracture fragments to help optimize presurgical planning (Fig. 8.8).

3D printing with biocompatible materials can be utilized internally as surgical hardware, external fixation and assistive devices, or as therapy-impregnated implants. Custom fabrication of PSI for routine joint total arthroplasty can improve alignment and reduce intraoperative time (Renson et al. 2014), although a few investigators report no significant improvement or added benefit in routine cases (Voleti et al. 2014; Sassoon et al. 2014). PSI is extremely useful in patients needing nonstandard joint replacement, joint replacement in unconventional anatomy, customized fixation hardware after surgical resection, and

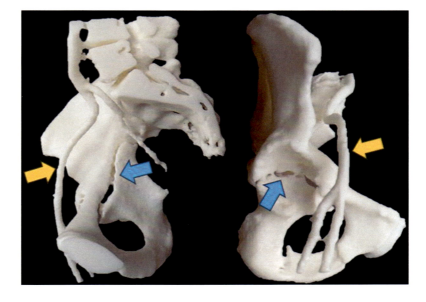

Fig. 8.8 3D model of complex acetabular fracture (*blue arrows*) involving anterior and posterior column and inferior pubic ramus. Fusion with CT angiography dataset enabled visualization of the relationship of the fracture with iliac vessels (*yellow arrows*)

patients with significant loss of bone stock after tumor resection. Customized hardware in such patients optimizes fixation biomechanics, thereby increasing stability and decreasing postoperative complications like hardware failure, implant collapse, and subsequent fracture risk. In total hip arthroplasty, for cases of extreme femoral medullary canal narrowing or abnormal anatomic axis of the femoral diaphysis, utilizing 3D printing for fabrication of the custom prosthetic femoral component and the receiving native femoral bone decreases risk of failed prosthetic insertion and intraoperative periprosthetic fracture (Faur et al. 2013). Newer patient-specific ceramic molds allow orthopedic implants to be casted out of a high-resistance cobalt-chrome alloy with built-in submillimeter integral bone ingrowth surface macro-textures which improve bone ingrowth fixation (Curodeau et al. 2000).

3D printed implants made of titanium alloy powder and porous implants have been used to reconstruct multilevel cervical spine in the setting of Ewing's sarcoma and metastatic papillary carcinoma with good success (Xu et al. 2016; Li et al. 2017). Customized acetabular implant specific to the patient and defect is termed a "tri-flange" which facilitates precise restoration of acetabular anatomy and hip biomechanics in patients with complex multiple revisions with poor bone stock and pelvis discontinuity (Wyatt 2015). Pelvic implants have been used for complex fractures (Mai et al. 2017) and following complex tumor resections (Wong et al. 2015).

In extremities, customized implants can be used in case of extensive resection or periarticular involvement. Suitable 3D printed endoprostheses can be created using patient-specific mirror image CT data from the normal contralateral extremity (Pruksakorn et al. 2014). Hollow 3D printed calcaneal prosthesis made of titanium has been used after a total calcanectomy for calcaneal chondrosarcoma allowing intraoperative reattachment of the Achilles tendon and the plantar fascia helping patient to become fully weight bearing and mobile in 5 months (Imanishi and Choong 2015). Scaphoid and lunate fractures are the two most common carpal bones affected by avascular necrosis due to limited vascularity

(Freedman et al. 2001). The possibility of 3D printed scaphoid and lunate bones with photocurable polymer would allow for implantation of the 3D printed carpal bones with suitable geometry, mechanical properties, and cytocompatibility for in vivo use (Gittard et al. 2009), avoiding other more invasive and extensive surgical options.

3D printing can address current challenges of external prosthetic development including high costs and limited availability. Pediatric prosthetic needs are complex owing to their small size, low weight requirement, constant need for size changes, and subsequent higher cost. In pediatric transradial amputees, 3D printed robotic prosthetics are lightweight and allow individual thumb movement with the ability to grasp objects with all five fingers (Gretsch et al. 2016). A major advantage the ease in scalability of the hand and socket model, allowing uncomplicated printing of new devices, as the patient ages (Fig. 8.9). Such prosthesis can be also be designed and printed remotely where detailed measurements can be extracted from photographs (Zuniga et al. 2015).

3D printed patient-specific external fixation hardware aids in treatment of fractures with accurate reduction, stable fixation, and strong anti-rotation and anti-bending abilities that prevent shear and rotational forces (Qiao et al. 2016). In addition to complex external devices, 3D printing can also be used to fashion routine splints in unconventional resource-constrained locations, for example, during space missions (Wong 2015). 3D printed patient-specific casts are superior to traditional casts as they have a lightweight ventilated structure and minimize distortion (Lin et al. 2016).

An interesting area of research development is drug-impregnated 3D implants which can provide both structural support and sustained local drug release to target locations. This has been utilized in the treatment of spinal tuberculosis using 3D printed macro-/mesoporous composite scaffold in which high doses of isoniazid and rifampin were loaded into chemically modified mesoporous bioactive ceramics and then bound with poly (3-hydroxybutyrate-co-3-hydroxyhexanoate) through a 3D printing procedure (Zhu et al. 2015). 3D porous scaffold

Fig. 8.9 3D printed low-cost pediatric prosthetic hand

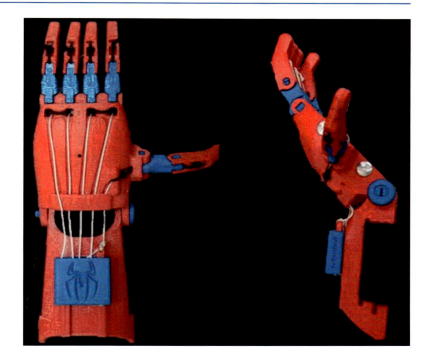

biomaterials have also been created by combining orthopedic reconstruction materials poly-DL-lactide and nano-hydroxyapatite with anti-TB medications (Dong et al. 2013). As this technology continues to evolve, there is potential for innovative patient-specific, disease-targeted, implantable 3D printed devices to treat other pathologies including neoplastic, metabolic, and endocrine disorders.

Areas of 3D musculoskeletal research and development continue to evolve. Tissue scaffolding and engineering are being increasingly used to promote cellular growth on a stable, patient-specific 3D printed framework. These scaffolds act as a support system where specific cellular tissue is subsequently implanted. The seeded scaffold can then be implanted at the desired site to promote cellular growth, remodeling, and regeneration. Scaffolds fabricated with 3D printing are reproducible, whereas native scaffolds may not be always readily available or reproduced (Grayson et al. 2009). In 3D printed scaffolds, the material properties, shape, bioactivity, and porosity can be customized for bone and cartilage regeneration.

For bone regeneration, custom-built 3D printed scaffolds derived from patient-specific CT data utilizing polycaprolactone (PCL) seeded with human adipose-derived stem cells (hASCs) have been used (Temple et al. 2014). These highly specialized 3D printed scaffolds promoted induction of hASCs to form vasculature and bone. The addition of a three-phase nanocrystalline hydroxyapatite (HA) and carbon nanotubes (CNT) to a polymeric matrix of PCL to fabricate a 3D printed scaffold has been shown to create a composite with compressive strength similar to trabecular bone and can promote good cell adhesion with adequate electrical conductivity to accommodate electrical stimuli that can be introduced for bone healing purposes (Gonçalves et al. 2016).

For cartilage regeneration, biocompatible hydrogels or water-absorbable cross-linked networks have been fabricated with 3D printing on a scaffold of biomaterials such as PCL. This creates a cartilaginous matrix in which chondrocytes and stem cells are encapsulated within the alginate hydrogels and can remain viable and metabolically active after implantation (Kundu et al. 2015). This treatment has the potential to promote chondral regeneration in cartilage injuries. Nanocomposite 3D printed osteochondral scaffolds using osteoconductive nanocrystalline hydroxyapatite (nHA) and core shell poly(lactic-co-glycolic) acid (PLGA) nanospheres encapsulated with chondrogenic transforming β1 (TGF-β1) improve human bone marrow-derived mesenchymal stem cell adhesion, proliferation, and osteochondral differentiation in biomimetic graded 3D printed osteochondral construct in vitro (Castro et al. 2015).

3D *organ* printing is a method of creating complex tissues by processing multiple biomaterials and cell types simultaneously. The musculoskeletal system presents a complex challenge in organ printing due to the biological and mechanical heterogeneity of tissues that are interfaced and work together to enact biomechanical function. The muscle-tendon unit (MTU), for example, is made up of three distinct regions with different properties: an elastic muscle that can relax and contract, a binding muscle-tendon junction, and a tendon with tensile properties. Merceron et al. (2015) report utilizing four components to create and integrate MTU tissue with regionally defined biological and mechanical properties.

3D models can provide numerous benefits although a few associated limitations need to be borne in mind. Postprocessing smoothing algorithms can mask fine details of patient's anatomy while resolving submillimetric pathology. Technical limitations of the 3D printer affect fidelity, with achievable spatial resolution usually of the order of 0.5 mm. Such minor imperfections, however, are usually clinically acceptable. Cost of printing a model may seem prohibitive; but the current printing cost of one presurgical model (excluding setup, installation, printer, and software costs) is under $100 and is expected to become less expensive in the future. The time required to print a model is in the order of a few hours, thereby prohibiting use in emergent surgical procedures. Nevertheless, technology and experience with 3D printing is rapidly evolving, and with further innovation, many of these limitations will be likely addressed in the near future.

With the rapid pace of innovation in 3D printing, the treatment and management of musculoskeletal pathology has continued to evolve. Handheld 3D models provide enhanced educational experience for the student, patient, and surgical team. Increased availability of 3D printing has shown substantial utility in preoperative planning and in the fabrication of custom implants and therapeutic devices. Cellular growth and regeneration with 3D printed scaffolds is an exciting area of continuing research and development with numerous potential applications.

References

Bagaria V, Deshpande S, Rasalkar DD, Kuthe A, Paunipagar BK. Use of rapid prototyping and three-dimensional reconstruction modeling in the management of complex fractures. Eur J Radiol. 2011;80(3):814–20.

Bellanova L, Paul L, Docquier PL. Surgical guides (patient-specific instruments) for pediatric tibial bone sarcoma resection and allograft reconstruction. Sarcoma. 2013;2013:787653.

Bizzotto N, Sandri A, Regis D, Romani D, Tami I, Magnan B. Three-dimensional printing of bone fractures. Surg Innov. 2015;22(5):548–51.

Bizzotto N, Tami I, Santucci A, Adani R, Poggi P, Romani D, et al. 3D printed replica of articular fractures for surgical planning and patient consent: a two years multi-centric experience. 3D Print Med. 2016a;2(1):2.

Bizzotto N, Tami I, Tami A, Spiegel A, Romani D, Corain M, et al. 3D printed models of distal radius fractures. Injury. 2016b;47(4):976–8.

Blakeney WG, Day R, Cusick L, Smith RL. Custom osteotomy guides for resection of a pelvic chondrosarcoma. Acta Orthop. 2014;85(4):438–41.

Brown GA, Firoozbakhsh K, DeCoster TA, Reyna JR Jr, Moneim M. Rapid prototyping: the future of trauma surgery? J Bone Joint Surg Am. 2003;85-A(Suppl 4):49–55.

Cartiaux O, Paul L, Francq BG, Banse X, Docquier PL. Improved accuracy with 3D planning and patient-specific instruments during simulated pelvic bone tumor surgery. Ann Biomed Eng. 2014;42(1):205–13.

Castro NJ, O'Brien J, Zhang LG. Integrating biologically inspired nanomaterials and table-top stereolithography for 3D printed biomimetic osteochondral scaffolds. Nanoscale. 2015;7(33):14010–22.

Chen S, Pan Z, Wu Y, Gu Z, Li M, Liang Z, et al. The role of three-dimensional printed models of skull in anatomy education: a randomized controlled trail. Sci Rep. 2017;7(1):575.

Curodeau A, Sachs E, Caldarise S. Design and fabrication of cast orthopedic implants with freeform surface textures from 3-D printed ceramic shell. J Biomed Mater Res. 2000;53(5):525–35.

Dong J, Zhang S, Liu H, Li X, Liu Y, Du Y. Novel alternative therapy for spinal tuberculosis during surgery: reconstructing with anti-tuberculosis bioactivity implants. Expert Opin Drug Deliv. 2013;11(3):299–305.

Faur C, Crainic N, Sticlaru C, Oancea C. Rapid prototyping technique in the preoperative planning for total hip arthroplasty with custom femoral components. Wien Klin Wochenschr. 2013;125(5–6):144–9.

Freedman DM, Botte MJ, Gelberman RH. Vascularity of the carpus. Clin Orthop Relat Res. 2001;(383):47–59.

Giovinco NA, Dunn SP, Dowling L, Smith C, Trowell L, Ruch JA, et al. A novel combination of printed 3-dimensional anatomic templates and computer-assisted surgical simulation for virtual preoperative planning in Charcot foot reconstruction. J Foot Ankle Surg. 2012;51(3):387–93.

Gittard SD, Narayan R, Lusk J, Morel P, Stockmans F, Ramsey M, et al. Rapid prototyping of scaphoid and lunate bones. Biotechnol J. 2009;4(1):129–34.

Gonçalves EM, Oliveira FJ, Silva RF, Neto MA, Fernandes MH, Amaral M, et al. Three-dimensional printed PCL-hydroxyapatite scaffolds filled with CNTs for bone cell growth stimulation. J Biomed Mater Res B Appl Biomater. 2016;104(6):1210–9.

Grayson WL, Frohlich M, Yeager K, Bhumiratana S, Chan ME, Cannizzaro C, et al. Engineering anatomically shaped human bone grafts. Proc Natl Acad Sci U S A. 2009;107(8):3299–304.

Gretsch KF, Lather HD, Peddada KV, Deeken CR, Wall LB, Goldfarb CA. Development of novel 3D-printed robotic prosthetic for transradial amputees. Prosthetics Orthot Int. 2016;40(3):400–3.

Guitton TG, Brouwer K, Lindenhovius AL, Dyer G, Zurakowski D, Mudgal CS, et al. Diagnostic accuracy of two-dimensional and three-dimensional imaging and modeling of radial head fractures. J Hand Microsurg. 2014;6(1):13–7.

Hedequist DJ, Emans JB. The correlation of preoperative three-dimensional computed tomography reconstructions with operative findings in congenital scoliosis. Spine. 2003;28(22):2531–4.

Hurson C, Tansey A, O'Donnchadha B, Nicholson P, Rice J, McElwain J. Rapid prototyping in the assessment, classification and preoperative planning of acetabular fractures. Injury. 2007;38(10):1158–62.

Imanishi J, Choong PFM. Three-dimensional printed calcaneal prosthesis following total calcanectomy. Int J Surg Case Rep. 2015;10:83–7.

Jun Y. Morphological analysis of the human knee joint for creating custom-made implant models. Int J Adv Manuf Technol. 2010;52(9–12):841–53.

Kang SJ, Oh MJ, Jeon SP. A novel and easy approach for contouring surgery in patients with craniofacial fibrous dysplasia. J Craniofac Surg. 2015;26(6):1977–8.

Krishnan SP, Dawood A, Richards R, Henckel J, Hart AJ. A review of rapid prototyped surgical guides for patient-specific total knee replacement. Bone Joint J. 2012;94-B(11):1457–61.

Kundu J, Shim J-H, Jang J, Kim S-W, Cho D-W. An additive manufacturing-based PCL-alginate-chondrocyte bioprinted scaffold for cartilage tissue engineering. J Tissue Eng Regen Med. 2015;9(11):1286–97.

Li H, Wang L, Mao Y, Wang Y, Dai K, Zhu Z. Revision of complex acetabular defects using cages with the aid of rapid prototyping. J Arthroplast. 2013;28(10):1770–5.

Li B, Chen B, Zhang Y, Wang X, Wang F, Xia H, et al. Comparative use of the computer-aided angiography and rapid prototyping technology versus conventional imaging in the management of the Tile C pelvic fractures. Int Orthop. 2015;40(1):161–6.

Li X, Wang Y, Zhao Y, Liu J, Xiao S, Mao K. Multi-level 3D printing implant for reconstructing cervical spine with metastatic papillary thyroid carcinoma. Spine (Phila Pa 1976). 2017 May 11; doi:10.1097/BRS.0000 000000002229Spine.

Lin H, Shi L, Wang D. A rapid and intelligent designing technique for patient-specific and 3D-printed orthopedic cast. 3D Print Med. 2016;2(1) doi:10.1186/s41205-016-0007-7.

Ma L, Zhou Y, Zhu Y, Lin Z, Wang Y, Zhang Y, et al. 3D-printed guiding templates for improved osteosarcoma resection. Sci Rep. 2016;6:23335.

Mahaisavariya B, Sitthiseripratip K, Oris P, Tongdee T. Rapid prototyping model for surgical planning of corrective osteotomy for cubitus varus: report of two cases. Injury Extra. 2006;37(5):176–80.

Mai JG, Gu C, Lin XZ, Li T, Huang WQ, Wang H, et al. Application of three-dimensional printing personalized acetabular wing-plate in treatment of complex acetabular fractures via lateral-rectus approach. Zhonghua Wai Ke Za Zhi. 2017;55(3):172–8.

Makinen TJ, Fichman SG, Watts E, Kuzyk PRT, Safir OA, Gross AE. The role of cages in the management of severe acetabular bone defects at revision arthroplasty. Bone Joint J. 2016;98-B(1_Supple_A):73–7.

Manganaro MS, Morag Y, Weadock WJ, Yablon CM, Gaetke-Udager K, Stein EB. Creating three-dimensional printed models of acetabular fractures for use as educational tools. Radiographics. 2017;37(3):871–80.

Mao K, Wang Y, Xiao S, Liu Z, Zhang Y, Zhang X, et al. Clinical application of computer-designed polystyrene models in complex severe spinal deformities: a pilot study. Eur Spine J. 2010;19(5):797–802.

McMenamin PG, Quayle MR, McHenry CR, Adams JW. The production of anatomical teaching resources using three-dimensional (3D) printing technology. Anat Sci Educ. 2014;7(6):479–86.

Merceron TK, Burt M, Seol Y-J, Kang H-W, Lee SJ, Yoo JJ, et al. A 3D bioprinted complex structure for engineering the muscle–tendon unit. Biofabrication. 2015;7(3):035003.

Minns RJ, Bibb R, Banks R, Sutton RA. The use of a reconstructed three-dimensional solid model from CT to aid the surgical management of a total knee arthroplasty: a case study. Med Eng Phys. 2003;25(6):523–6.

Mizutani J, Matsubara T, Fukuoka M, Tanaka N, Iguchi H, Furuya A, et al. Application of full-scale three-dimensional models in patients with rheumatoid cervical spine. Eur Spine J. 2008;17(5):644–9.

Peters P, Langlotz F, Nolte LP. Computer assisted screw insertion into real 3D rapid prototyping pelvis models. Clin Biomech (Bristol, Avon). 2002;17(5):376–82.

Pruksakorn D, Chantarapanich N, Arpornchayanon O, Leerapun T, Sitthiseripratip K, Vatanapatimakul N. Rapid-prototype endoprosthesis for palliative reconstruction of an upper extremity after resection of bone metastasis. Int J Comput Assist Radiol Surg. 2014;10(3):343–50.

Qiao F, Li D, Jin Z, Hao D, Liao Y, Gong S. A novel combination of computer-assisted reduction technique and three dimensional printed patient-specific external fixator for treatment of tibial fractures. Int Orthop. 2016;40(4):835–41.

Renson L, Poilvache P, Van den Wyngaert H. Improved alignment and operating room efficiency with patient-specific instrumentation for TKA. Knee. 2014;21(6):1216–20.

Sassoon A, Nam D, Nunley R, Barrack R. Systematic review of patient-specific instrumentation in total knee arthroplasty: new but not improved. Clin Orthop Relat Res. 2014;473(1):151–8.

Schwartz A, Money K, Spangehl M, Hattrup S, Claridge RJ, Beauchamp C. Office-based rapid prototyping in orthopedic surgery: a novel planning technique and review of the literature. Am J Orthop (Belle Mead NJ). 2015;44(1):19–25.

Sheth U, Theodoropoulos J, Abouali J. Use of 3-dimensional printing for preoperative planning in the treatment of recurrent anterior shoulder instability. Arthrosc Tech. 2015;4(4):e311–6.

Starosolski ZA, Kan JH, Rosenfeld SD, Krishnamurthy R, Annapragada A. Application of 3-D printing (rapid prototyping) for creating physical models of pediatric orthopedic disorders. Pediatr Radiol. 2013;44(2):216–21.

Subburaj K, Ravi B, Agarwal M. Automated identification of anatomical landmarks on 3D bone models reconstructed from CT scan images. Comput Med Imaging Graph. 2009;33(5):359–68.

Tack P, Victor J, Gemmel P, Annemans L. 3D-printing techniques in a medical setting: a systematic literature review. Biomed Eng Online. 2016;15(1):115.

Tam MD, Laycock SD, Bell D, Chojnowski A. 3-D print-out of a DICOM file to aid surgical planning in a 6 year old patient with a large scapular osteochondroma complicating congenital diaphyseal aclasia. J Radiol Case Rep. 2012;6(1):31–7.

Temple JP, Hutton DL, Hung BP, Huri PY, Cook CA, Kondragunta R, et al. Engineering anatomically shaped vascularized bone grafts with hASCs and 3D-printed PCL scaffolds. J Biomed Mater Res A. 2014;102(12):4317–25.

Upex P, Jouffroy P, Riouallon G. Application of 3D printing for treating fractures of both columns of the acetabulum: benefit of pre-contouring plates on the mirrored healthy pelvis. Orthop Traumatol Surg Res. 2017;103(3):331–4.

Voleti PB, Hamula MJ, Baldwin KD, Lee G-C. Current data do not support routine use of patient-specific instrumentation in total knee arthroplasty. J Arthroplast. 2014;29(9):1709–12.

West SJ, Mari JM, Khan A, Wan JH, Zhu W, Koutsakos IG, et al. Development of an ultrasound phantom for spinal injections with 3-dimensional printing. Reg Anesth Pain Med. 2014;39(5):429–33.

Won SH, Lee YK, Ha YC, Suh YS, Koo KH. Improving pre-operative planning for complex total hip replacement with a rapid prototype model enabling surgical simulation. Bone Joint J. 2013;95-B(11):1458–63.

Wong JY. On-site 3D printing of functional custom mallet splints for Mars analogue crewmembers. Aerosp Med Hum Perform. 2015;86(10):911–4.

Wong KC, Kumta SM, Chiu KH, Antonio GE, Unwin P, Leung KS. Precision tumour resection and reconstruction using image-guided computer navigation. J Bone Joint Surg Br. 2007a;89(7):943–7.

Wong KC, Kumta SM, Chiu KH, Cheung KW, Leung KS, Unwin P, et al. Computer assisted pelvic tumor resection and reconstruction with a custom-made prosthesis using an innovative adaptation and its validation. Comput Aided Surg. 2007b;12(4):225–32.

Wong KC, Kumta SM, Geel NV, Demol J. One-step reconstruction with a 3D-printed, biomechanically evaluated custom implant after complex pelvic tumor resection. Comput Aided Surg. 2015;20(1):14–23.

Wu Z-X, Huang L-Y, Sang H-X, Ma Z-S, Wan S-Y, Cui G, et al. Accuracy and safety assessment of pedicle screw placement using the rapid prototyping technique in severe congenital scoliosis. J Spinal Disord Tech. 2011;24(7):444–50.

Wu XB, Wang JQ, Zhao CP, Sun X, Shi Y, Zhang ZA, et al. Printed three-dimensional anatomic templates for virtual preoperative planning before reconstruction of old pelvic injuries: initial results. Chin Med J. 2015;128(4):477–82.

Wyatt MC. Custom 3D-printed acetabular implants in hip surgery – innovative breakthrough or expensive bespoke upgrade? Hip Int. 2015;25(4):375–9.

Xiao J-R, Huang W-D, Yang X-H, Yan W-J, Song D-W, Wei H-F, et al. En bloc resection of primary malignant bone tumor in the cervical spine based on 3-dimensional printing technology. Orthop Surg. 2016;8(2):171–8.

Xu N, Wei F, Liu X, Jiang L, Cai H, Li Z, et al. Reconstruction of the upper cervical spine using a personalized 3D-printed vertebral body in an adolescent with Ewing sarcoma. Spine. 2016;41(1):E50–4.

Zeng C, Xing W, Wu Z, Huang H, Huang W. A combination of three-dimensional printing and computer-assisted virtual surgical procedure for preoperative planning of acetabular fracture reduction. Injury. 2016;47(10):2223–7.

Zhu M, Li K, Zhu Y, Zhang J, Ye X. 3D-printed hierarchical scaffold for localized isoniazid/rifampin drug delivery and osteoarticular tuberculosis therapy. Acta Biomater. 2015;16:145–55.

Zuniga J, Katsavelis D, Peck J, Stollberg J, Petrykowski M, Carson A, et al. Cyborg beast: a low-cost 3d-printed prosthetic hand for children with upper-limb differences. BMC Res Notes. 2015;8(1):10.

3D Printing and Patient-Matched Implants

9

Andrew M. Christensen

9.1 Background

Patient-matched implants were one of the first great applications of 3D printing in medicine (Mankovich et al. 1990; Stoker et al. 1992; Binder and Kaye 1994; Komori et al. 1994). Even preceding the advent of 3D printing, surgeons were using crude, more manually constructed models to aid in design of a patient-matched implant for some of the most complex reconstructive surgeries, surgeries such as for reconstruction of pelvic discontinuity following tumor removal. An anatomical model which clearly displays the deficit one is trying to reconstruct is a perfect application. Reported benefits for prefabricated implants include surgical time savings, ease of adaptation in surgery, perfected shape or design, and an ability to reconstruct anatomical areas that have no other alternatives from an implant standpoint (Hamid et al. 2016; McAloon 1997; Erickson et al. 1999; Taunton et al. 2012). In many of the initial cases, 3D printing was not used to create the actual implant, but instead it helped to facilitate the design, workflow, or manufacturing of tools used to create these implants. Surgeon adaptation of plates using an anatomical model is also tangentially related to the topic of patient-matched implants. This very "manual" technique for personalizing an implant has been a mainstay of medical modeling since the earliest days (Eppley and Sadove 1998) (Figs. 9.1 and 9.2).

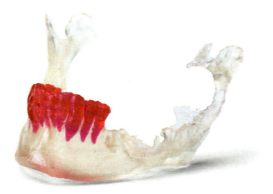

Fig. 9.1 Stereolithography model of a patient with a left mandibular tumor which has eaten away the bone. Surgery will involve removing almost half of the mandible and replacing with a large reconstruction plate and bone graft. Courtesy 3D Systems, Rock Hill, South Carolina, USA

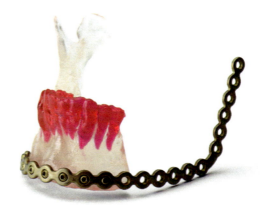

Fig. 9.2 The surgical removal of the left mandible has been simulated and a titanium reconstruction plate has been pre-bent before surgery. Performing the bending before surgery both saves time in surgery and provides for a better aesthetic outcome for the patient. Courtesy 3D Systems, Rock Hill, South Carolina, USA

A.M. Christensen
SOMADEN LLC, 8156 S. Wadsworth Blvd., Unit E-357, Littleton, CO 80128, USA
e-mail: biomdlr@me.com

© Springer International Publishing AG 2017
F.J. Rybicki, G.T. Grant (eds.), *3D Printing in Medicine*, DOI 10.1007/978-3-319-61924-8_9

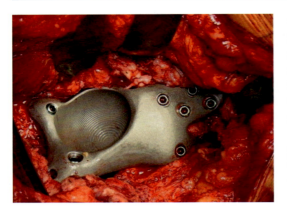

Fig. 9.3 Patient-matched acetabular cup produced by 3D printing shown during surgical insertion. Courtesy P. James Burn, MD and Paul Morrison, Ossis Ltd., Christchurch, New Zealand

In the last 5 years, the direct output of implantable parts produced using 3D printing has become more common (Hamid et al. 2016; Di Prima et al. 2016). When 3D printing is directly used for output of a patient-matched implant, it takes advantage of the fact that one-off designs are suited very well to this manufacturing technique. Another benefit of 3D printing is that "complexity is free," and many times the more complex the design is, the faster and more economical the design is to actually produce (Fig. 9.3). This is a major shift in terms of design thinking, where biomedical engineers and others who have produced implants traditionally using subtractive machining need to reorient and expand their design thinking, which often adds constraints imposed by manufacturing processes.

In the 1990s, early uses for patient-matched implants centered around craniomaxillofacial (CMF) applications; and these are still likely the most prevalent by percentage of total cases in any one anatomical area (Chepelev et al. 2017). Based on the intrinsic complexity of the face and the need for not only functional but aesthetic reconstruction, CMF applications continue to be solid users of patient-matched implant technology (Erickson et al. 1999; Powers et al. 1998; Müller et al. 2003). The technology matured in other areas of the body for large reconstructive surgery cases, many of which were oncology cases (Mulford et al. 2016). Over time, many more applications arose such as limb salvage procedures where complexity is created with defects that are not easily reconstructed with off-the-shelf sizes or shapes of implants. 3D printing is advantageous for the creation of patient-matched implants due to its accurate shape and scale, as well as the ability to print contralateral anatomy to use as a reference for anatomical reconstruction.

Currently, there is a major shift away from patient-matched implants being used solely for the extreme, massive reconstructive surgery cases toward these technologies being used for more "everyday" types of surgical cases. For example, one area that is now largely patient-matched is cranioplasty for repair of large cranial defects. For a defect over a couple of inches in diameter, a very large number of these neurosurgery cases worldwide involve prefabrication of a cranioplasty implant powered by 3D printing technology (Roberson and Rosenberg 1997; Eppley and Sadove 1998). Other even more common areas such as knee replacement are now also beginning to catch on, with patient-matched implant workflows being more commonly offered for partial or total knee arthroplasty (Slamin and Parsley 2012).

9.2 Terminology

From a regulatory standpoint, the terminology used to describe a patient-specific implant is important. Historically, the word "custom" has been used to describe 3D printed implants made for a specific patient using medical image data. However, from the US FDA's perspective, the term "custom" is closely affiliated with the Custom Device Exemption (FDA 2014), a very specific, defined regulatory path for use of a singular device in the treatment of a singular patient. Such devices have many restrictions, the most major of which is that no other commercially available device is available to treat the patient's condition. Other major drawbacks to using the Custom Device Exemption for provision of an implant, from a device manufacturer's standpoint, are related to the fact that there is a strict five units per year limit and that no marketing may be performed, both which severely hinder the ability to provide implants on a widespread basis under the Custom Device Exemption.

The FDA has recommended the use of the terminology "patient-matched" in an effort to make more clear the delineation between devices which go through a rigorous marketing clearance process such as a 510(k) or Premarket Approval (PMA), patient-matched, and those which are used on more of a one-off basis for a truly unique surgical situation, custom devices (FDA 2016). Patient-matched implants going through the FDA's traditional regulatory pathways for marketing clearance are much like regular, off-the-shelf-sized implants; however, instead of the FDA clearing the implant size, shape, etc., the FDA is clearing the "system" of design which leads to the final design. The system concept would talk about the inputs such as medical imaging studies and design constraints. The final design must fit into a bounding box that the company determines up front, allowing for testing at the extents of thickness, size, expanse, and material, among other considerations.

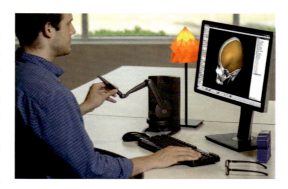

Fig. 9.4 An engineer uses Geomagic Freeform software to design a patient-matched cranioplasty. The tool in his left hand provides force feedback, giving the designer the sensation of "touching" the design he is working on. Courtesy 3D Systems, Rock Hill, South Carolina, USA

9.3 Medical Imaging and Digital Design of Patient-Matched Implants

Modern volumetric medical imaging studies can produce high-quality images that are usable for patient-matched implants. Most implants made for reconstruction of bony anatomy are designed with the aid of preoperative computed tomography (CT) scans. Typical workflows for medical image processing to extract the exact area of anatomy in question are performed by qualified technicians using specialized software tools. When the anatomy in question has been segmented, the workflow can proceed in a number of different ways depending on the patient-matched implant needs. This could look as simple as an anatomical model being 3D printed or as complex as a manufacturing mold being output or even direct output of the implant via 3D printing in a biocompatible material.

Although medical imaging has long been ready to support patient-matched implants, the software tools for digital design of the implants themselves have not always been robust enough for these tasks. It was only following the year 2000 that software tools which would allow for precise manipulation of very organic shapes became available. Many of those tools are still widely used today for implant design, tools such as Geomagic Freeform (3D Systems, Rock Hill, SC). Freeform is somewhat unique in that it combines organic manipulation software with haptic feedback, so the user can actually "feel" the model they are working on in digital space (Fig. 9.4). For many patient-specific implants which are anatomically designed (i.e., meant to mimic the shape of the anatomy they are replacing), this tool has been incredibly powerful. Other design tasks in different industries like the footwear industry also rely heavily on organic modeling software, which can be used to design very complex geometries for things like shoe soles. Digital design is most powerful in designing net-shape (final, perfect design) designs which can be directly built using digital fabrication techniques like 3D printing. In addition, digital design can also be used to design near-net-shape (close to final design) parts for surgeon input, further design, and rough design iterations.

This is an exciting time for patient-matched implants from a design software standpoint. In the past, only very "one-off" implants were created with 3D printing, and these were primarily designed by hand, even when a designer would do this work digitally. Today the tools exist to almost totally automate many of these design tasks, taking what has been labor intensive and making it effortless once the system is developed. In addition to saving time and money on labor, other benefits of automation of design include reproducibility and standardization, both of which are much more predictable with automation of design. Watch this space for the coming 5 years to see automation totally change the economics and timeframes and accessibility of truly personalized, patient-matched design.

9.4   How 3D Printing Fits In

There is no single tool or method that fits the needs for all types of patient-matched implants. 3D printing supports the creation of patient-matched implants in a variety of ways including:

1. Anatomical model as a baseline for a design which is performed manually (i.e., with wax or clay)
2. Anatomical model as a template for preparing an off-the shelf implant by hand during or before surgery
3. Different types of models as manufacturing tools following digital design of the implant (molds for forming materials or sacrificial wax patterns)
4. Digital design and 3d printed fabrication of these implants directly in an implantable biomaterial

1. *Anatomical Models as Baseline for Manual Design*
   In this scenario, the anatomical model is 3D printed and is used for the surgeon and engineer to develop an implant design. Many bone reconstructive, implantable devices have been designed in this way, allowing the surgeon to visualize the anatomy clearly in hand and to make needed modifications to the anatomy such as removing bone spurs and existing implants before design of a patient-matched implant (Fig. 9.5). The design of the implant could be as simple as creating a wax pattern of the implant on the model. Later this design could be investment cast into metal, machined

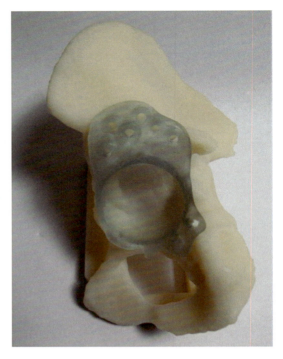

Fig. 9.5 A 3D printed trial implant (*blue green*) on a patient-specific bone model for a patient-matched hip reconstruction case. Courtesy P. James Burn, MD and Paul Morrison, Ossis Ltd., Christchurch, New Zealand

by tracer mill, or digitized for computer numerical control (CNC) machining. Historically, without digital design tools, this has been the most common method to create a patient-matched implant; however, given the tools today available for digital design, this method has been surpassed by these more digital techniques.

2. *Intraoperative or Immediately Preoperative Bending/Fitting by Surgeons*
   Many times models or templates are used to create patient-matched implants by the surgeon doing the fabrication using the model and the implant (think of a reconstruction plate being bent). This is also very common for personalizing implant hardware which is fairly straightforward and easy for the surgeon to modify in fitting to the patient's anatomy.
3. *Models as a Manufacturing Tool/Pattern*
   If implant design is carried out digitally, there will be a need to output that design into physical form. Many methods exist, but the two main

methods include (a) the digital design of the implant is produced as a sacrificial pattern for investment casting and (b) the digital design is subtracted from a box and output as a two-part mold for injection molding of the implant.

(a) *Sacrificial Pattern 3D Printing of the Implant Design.* In this scenario, one could imagine a proximal total knee component being digitally designed with the target material being cobalt-chrome (Co-Cr) alloy. Co-Cr is typically investment cast for these applications using a sacrificial wax pattern invested in plaster. In this case, the digitally designed, patient-matched implant is 3D printed in wax or another investment casting-friendly material. Once printed, the pattern is used in the more traditional workflow for investment casting and subsequent finishing and polishing of the implant.

(b) *3D Printing of a Mold for Injection Molding.* In this scenario, the implant may be polymeric and in a material that is not yet easy to directly 3D print. The net-shape designed implant would be digitally subtracted from a box, which would then be cut to form a two-part mold, with a cavity inside where the implant would be formed. Sprues and channels can be added to the digital model before being 3D printed in a material conducive to injection molding of the final implant material. Once the mold is 3D printed, the injection molding (i.e., injecting material into the mold to form the shape of the implant) is completed, and the implant is finished, packaged, and readied for use. This method is common for implant materials which are not yet suited for direct 3D printing.

4. *Digital Design and 3D Printing of Implants Directly in an Implantable Material*

The most direct route to production of a patient-matched implant would be to directly 3D print it in a suitable biomaterial. Today there exist 3D printing techniques to produce implantable parts in various biocompatible metals and plastics. Most common direct metal applications are produced by powder bed fusion techniques (EBM, DMLS, SLM, DMP) in titanium, titanium alloys, and cobalt-chrome alloy. In polymers, most of the implantable work to date has been performed using laser sintering of polyether ether ketone (PEEK) and polyether ketone ketone (PEKK) materials, with others like silicone and polyethylene being researched. 3D printing of titanium and other implant biomaterials has been going on for the last 10+ years with the first FDA clearance for a titanium, 3D printed implant in 2010 (FDA 2010), and the first FDA clearance for a polymeric, 3D printed implant in 2013 (FDA 2013). Regardless of these approvals, many of the patient-matched implants created today are still produced by machining, investment casting, or injection molding versus 3D printing.

9.5 Patient-Matched Implant Examples

A few examples of patient-matched implants are included below for illustration of the scope of procedures benefitted and general use of 3D printing technology.

1. *Facial Augmentation with Silicone Implant.* Patients requiring augmentation of soft tissue or bony deformities of the face can benefit from the use of patient-matched silicone implants (Fig. 9.6). These implants may be designed by hand or digitally against the patient-matched bone model.

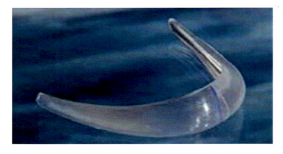

Fig. 9.6 Silicone genial implant for a patient requiring augmentation of the chin. Courtesy of Implantech Associates, Ventura, California, USA

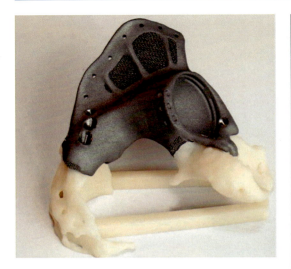

Fig. 9.7 Hemi-pelvic reconstruction using a patient-matched 3D printed titanium alloy implant. Note areas of the design which are porous for planned adhesion of tissue. Courtesy P. James Burn MD and Paul Morrison, Ossis Ltd., Christchurch, New Zealand

2. *Hemi-Pelvis Reconstruction with 3D Printed Titanium Implant*. Oncology patients often require substantial reconstruction following removal of large sections of cancerous tissue. Directly 3D printed titanium alloy implants (EBM, Powder Bed Fusion) combined with fully digital design take advantage of the ability of 3D printing to produce complex, organic shapes. Notice the porous section of the flange, specifically designed for greater muscle adhesion (Fig. 9.7).

3. *Revision Hip Arthroplasty*. Roughly 15% of all total hip arthroplasty procedures performed annually are revision procedures, with an increasing number of patients on their second or third revision. Each revision removes more of the good, baseline bone that is required for optimal fixation of the acetabular cup. When extensive bone loss is encountered, a patient-matched implant may be an optimal solution, designed for contact with the patient's anatomy in optimal locations. Direct production by 3D printing in titanium alloy (EBM, Powder Bed Fusion) is accomplished after the implant is digitally designed (Figs. 9.8 and 9.9).

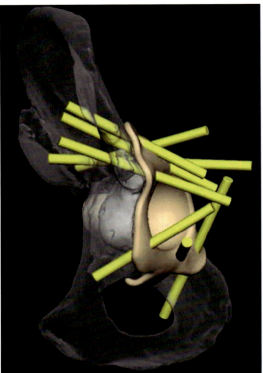

Fig. 9.8 Patient-matched design of a revision acetabular component allows for precise locating of screw trajectory and placement (*yellow*). Courtesy P. James Burn MD and Paul Morrison, Ossis Ltd., Christchurch, New Zealand

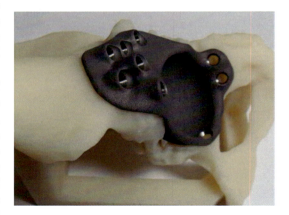

Fig. 9.9 Patient-matched 3D printed titanium implant for a patient requiring revision hip arthroplasty. Courtesy P. James Burn MD and Paul Morrison, Ossis Ltd., Christchurch, New Zealand

4. *Directly 3D Printed Cranioplasty in PEKK*. Direct output of implantable polymers with FDA clearance has only been available since

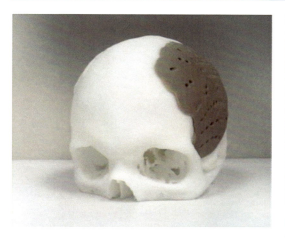

Fig. 9.10 Cranioplasty implant 3D printed in PEKK biomaterial for a patient with a large cranial defect. Courtesy Oxford Performance Materials, South Windsor, Connecticut, USA

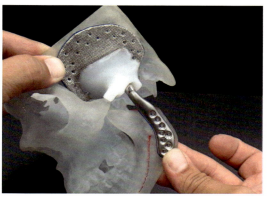

Fig. 9.11 Patient-matched total temporomandibular joint (TMJ) replacement with temporal extension covering a larger than normal defect. 3D printed model integral to the design and manufacturing process. Courtesy TMJ Concepts, Ventura, California, USA

2013. Oxford Performance Materials using their unique PEKK (polyether ketone ketone) biomaterial have paved the way in this area. In this example of a cranioplasty implant, the patient has a large defect in the skull, likely due to trauma or previous surgical intervention (Fig. 9.10). Digital design of the implant is carried out and direct 3D printing of the implant in PEKK biomaterial is performed (Laser Sintering, Powder Bed Fusion).

5. *TMJ and Mandibular Reconstruction.* One of the early, most common applications for patient-matched implants was in the area of total temporomandibular joint (TMJ) reconstruction (Worford et al. 2015). Many times the implants will be produced traditionally (i.e., CNC machined or formed without 3D printing), but the 3D printed anatomical model will be key to the process of personalizing the design (Fig. 9.11).

6. *Machined PEEK Zygoma Implants.* Personalized reconstructive facial prostheses like this zygoma plus orbital floor implant are gaining popularity in the plastic surgery and oral and maxillofacial surgical communities. Patients that have had a traumatic injury many times will require some augmentation to the bony structures to again regain their normal appearance. For some of these cases, the globe of the eye may also be

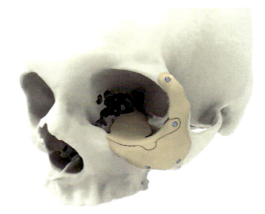

Fig. 9.12 Machined PEEK implants are produced by milling from a digital design. 3D printed anatomical models form a basis for the design and quality control of these components. Courtesy KLS Martin, Jacksonville, Florida, USA

in a suboptimal position. Using digital design and machining of PEEK (polyether ether ketone), these implants can be output utilizing a "puzzle-piece" design to allow for optimal stability after implantation (Fig. 9.12).

7. *Directly 3D Printed Titanium Mandibular Reconstruction Plate.* A fairly common application for digital planning and patient-matched implants are for mandibular reconstruction. In this case, the titanium plate is 3D printed in titanium (Laser Sintering, Powder Bed Fusion) for precise adaptation

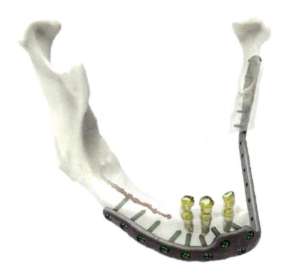

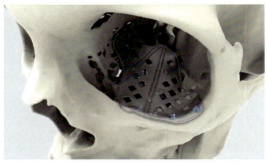

Fig. 9.14 A patient-matched orbital floor plate (*gray*) which has been designed based on the patient's CT scan and digitally output by 3D printing in titanium. Courtesy KLS Martin, Jacksonville, Florida, USA

Fig. 9.13 3D Printed mandibular reconstruction plate (*gray*) following a resection of the left mandible. Precise screw locations and contour can be achieved by the combination of digital design and digital output. Courtesy KLS Martin, Jacksonville, Florida, USA

to the desired shape of the mandible following resection of a portion of the mandible (Fig. 9.13).

8. *Patient-Matched Orbital Floor Implant.* Many times in facial fracture cases, the patient will suffer an orbital floor "blowout" whereby the thin bone of the floor of the orbit fractures and is displaced into the maxillary sinus, causing the globe to displace inferiorly. A patient-matched implant such as this 3D printed titanium (Laser Sintering, Powder Bed Fusion) implant will be used to perfectly repair the orbital floor while not impinging on other areas that are sensitive, such as the optic nerve (Fig. 9.14).

9. *Salvage Ankle Fusion Cage Directly 3D Printed in Titanium (Hamid et al. 2016).* There are many times that large defects threaten the viability of a limb from a stability and vascularity standpoint. Limb salvage procedures are there to save the limb from the possibility of amputation. In this case, the patient presented with a comminuted fracture of the ankle and was given several options, including amputation of the foot (Fig. 9.15). A patient-matched 3D printed

titanium (EBM, Powder Bed Fusion) cage was designed to allow her to keep her foot and to be used in conjunction with adjacent hardware (rod, screws).

10. *Distal Humeral Resurfacing Implant Directly 3D Printed in Titanium (Fig. 9.16).*

11. *3D Printed, Bioresorbable Tracheal Splint for Tracheobronchomalacia (Morrison et al. 2015).* A patient-matched, 3D printed tracheal splint was developed by the University of Michigan to treat young children with a rare condition called tracheobronchomalacia (TBM), a collapse of the airway. The splint is designed from the patient's CT scan of the airway using Materialise Mimics software and 3D printed out of a bioresorbable material. The intent is the splint will support the bronchus locally preventing airway collapse and will eventually resorb once the patient's airway has remodeled. The company Materialise and the University of Michigan are partnered to bring this breakthrough device and technology through to commercialization (Fig. 9.17).

Some of the examples shown are truly custom devices as discussed earlier when talking about terminology, and some are more commercially available, having gone through a more formal premarket clearance process [510(k) or PMA] with the US FDA.

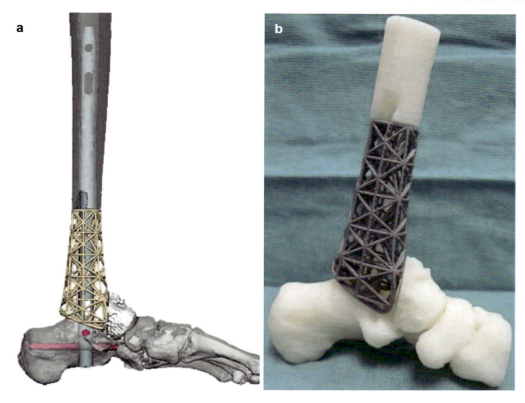

Fig. 9.15 (**a**) and (**b**) Large 3D printed titanium cage that was packed with bone graft to augment a missing area of anatomy in the lower leg just at the ankle. Courtesy 4WEB Medical, Frisco, Texas, USA

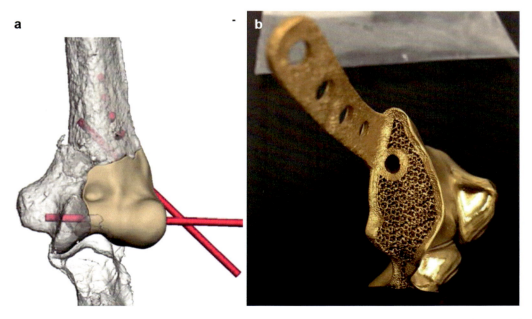

Fig. 9.16 (**a**) and (**b**) Distal humeral resurfacing implant produced by 3D printing in titanium with additional titanium nitride coating. Note the porous area for bone ingrowth and the highly polished joint surface area for articulation against the opposing, native bone. Courtesy 4WEB Medical, Frisco, Texas, USA

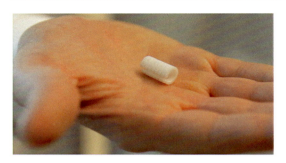

Fig. 9.17 A patient-matched, 3D printed tracheal splint was developed by the University of Michigan to treat young children with a rare condition called tracheobronchomalacia (TBM), a collapse of the airway. The splint is designed from the patient's CT scan of the airway using Materialise Mimics software and 3D printed out of a bioresorbable material. Courtesy Materialise USA, Plymouth, Michigan, USA and University of Michigan, Ann Arbor, Michigan, USA

9.6 Conclusions

Taking a survey today of the entire reconstructive implant industry spanning many specialties, one would find patient-matched implants being used more than ever before with applications spanning the entire body. There is a demonstrated utility for patient-matched implant technology when applying this to very uncommon and special reconstructive surgeries. Over time, though, a multitude of applications which are more common have arisen to make these personalized implants useful to a greater variety of patients. Mostly anecdotal reports of surgical time savings when using patient-matched implants have cemented their use for certain areas such as large oncologic reconstructions. Further study is ongoing to show that personalized implants applied to areas like total knee reconstruction can provide patient benefit in the long term, in addition to aiding the surgeon's technical job during surgery.

Personalized surgery is a growing topic and will guide further growth and infiltration into many areas where traditionally the "one size fits all" approach has been used. Key to the further widespread adoption of patient-matched technology will be that it is not only better for the patient and the surgeon but also better for the hospital and the payer who is footing the cost. Today when one mentions "patient-matched implants" relative to cost, there is a thought that patient-matched means expensive. Further software automation and better direct implant output via 3D printing will be part of the solution to push the expense for these devices down which will push down their prices. The future is bright for further adoption of patient-matched implant technology in many different areas of the body.

References

Binder WJ, Kaye AH. Three-dimensional computer modeling. Facial Plast Surg Clin North Am. 1994;2:357.

Chepelev L, Giannopoulos A, Tang A, et al. Medical 3D printing: methods to standardize terminology and report trends. 3D Print Med. 2017;3:4. doi:10.1186/s41205-017-0012-5.

Di Prima M, Coburn J, Hwang D, Kelly J, Khairuzzaman A, Ricles L. Additively manufactured medical products – the FDA perspective. 3D Print Med. 2016;2:1. doi:10.1186/s41205-016-0005-9.

Eppley BL, Sadove AM. Computer generated patient models for reconstruction of cranial and facial deformities. J Craniofac Surg. 1998;6:548.

Erickson DM, Chance D, Schmitt S, et al. An opinion survey of reported benefits from the use of stereolithographic models. J Oral Maxillofac Surg. 1999;57:1040.

FDA. Exactech 510(k) K102975 Exactech Novation Crown Cup with InteGrip acetabular shell. November 5, 2010. https://www.accessdata.fda.gov/cdrh_docs/pdf10/K102975.pdf. Accessed 2017 Apr 30.

FDA. Oxford performance materials 510(k) K121818 OsteoFab™ patient-specific cranial device. Feb 7, 2013. https://www.accessdata.fda.gov/cdrh_docs/pdf12/K121818.pdf. Accessed 2017 Apr 30.

FDA. Custom device exemption guidance for industry and FDA staff. Document issued on September 24, 2014. https://www.fda.gov/downloads/medicaldevices/deviceregulationandguidance/guidancedocuments/ucm415799.pdf. Accessed 2017 Apr 30.

FDA. Technical considerations for additive manufactured devices, draft guidance for industry and FDA Staff. May 10, 2016. https://www.fda.gov/downloads/MedicalDevices/DeviceRegulationandGuidance/GuidanceDocuments/UCM499809.pdf. Accessed 2017 Apr 30.

Hamid KS, Parekh SG, Adams SB. Salvage of severe foot and ankle trauma with a 3D printed scaffold. Foot Ankle Int. 2016;37(4):433–9.

Komori T, Takato T, Akagawa T. Use of a laser-hardened three-dimensional replica for simulated surgery. J Oral Maxillofac Surg. 1994;52:516.

Mankovich NJ, Cheeseman AM, Stoker NJ. The display of three-dimensional anatomy with stereolithographic models. J Digit Imaging. 1990;3:200.

McAloon K. Rapid prototyping technology: a unique approach to the diagnosis and planning of medical procedures. Dearborn, MI: The Society of Manufacturing Engineers; 1997.

Morrison RJ, Hollister SJ, Niedner MF, et al. Mitigation of tracheobronchomalacia with 3D-printed personalized medical devices in pediatric patients. Sci Transl Med. 2015;7:285ra64.

Mulford JS, Babazadeh S, Mackay N. Three-dimensional printing in orthopaedic surgery: review of current and future applications. ANZ J Surg. 2016;86(9):648–53.

Müller A, Krishnan KG, Uhl E, Mast G. The application of rapid prototyping techniques in cranial reconstruction and preoperative planning in neurosurgery. J Craniofac Surg. 2003;14:899–914.

Powers DB, Edgin WA, Tabatchnick L. Stereolithography: a historical review and indications for use in the management of trauma. J Craniomaxillofac Trauma. 1998;4:16.

Roberson JB, Rosenberg WS. Traumatic cranial defects reconstructed with the HTR-PMI cranioplastic implant. J Craniomaxillofac Trauma. 1997;3(2):8–13.

Slamin J, Parsley B. Evolution of customization design for total knee arthroplasty. Curr Rev Muscoskelet Med. 2012;5(4):290–5.

Stoker NG, Mankovich NJ, Valentino D. Stereolithographic models for surgical planning. J Oral Maxillofac Surg. 1992;50:466.

Taunton MJ, et al. Pelvic discontinuity treated with custom triflange component: a reliable option. Clin Orthop Relat Res. 2012;470(2):428–34.

FDA Regulatory Pathways and Technical Considerations for the 3D Printing of Medical Models and Devices

10

James C. Coburn and Gerald T. Grant

10.1 Introduction

The advances in medical imaging, application of interactive 3D design software, and advances in additive manufacturing techniques have provided an unprecedented opportunity for innovative and customized patient care. These advances are not only available to the commercial manufacturing of medical/dental devices, but by their very nature are scalable from institutions such as major medical centers to local medical and dental practices. In the past 15 years, the application of digital imaging, digital design, and digital manufacturing (both subtractive and additive) has proven to decrease operating times and provide better patient outcomes in areas where customized surgical (Fig. 10.1) and restorative plans were indicated. These results have in many cases simplified more complicated treatment options such as dental implant placement and restoration and provided the opportunity to design and fabricated complex structures for use emergent patient care, such as airway assist devices in pediatric patients. As the designer and manufacturer of these types of devices that are often part of an institution or a

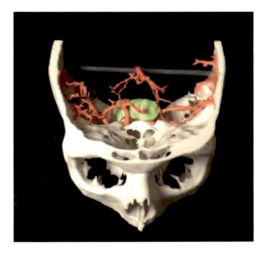

Fig. 10.1 Medical model of tumor and vasculature

private office, there are now individuals fabricating devices that may not be aware of possible regulation of devices or in some cases are reluctant to use this technology for the same reason.

The intent of this chapter is to familiarize the reader to the role of the FDA in medical device development and regulation and to hopefully clear up some misconceptions and provide guidance in the application of these technologies in patient care.

10.2 The FDA's Role

The FDA is charged with ensuring that medical products sold in the United States, including drugs, devices, and biologics, are safe and effective

J.C. Coburn, M.S., C.P.H. (✉)
US Food and Drug Administration,
Silver Spring, MD, USA
e-mail: james.coburn@fda.hhs.gov

G.T. Grant, D.M.D., M.S.
University of Louisville, School of Dentistry,
Louisville, KY, USA
e-mail: gerald.grant@louisville.edu

© Springer International Publishing AG 2017
F.J. Rybicki, G.T. Grant (eds.), *3D Printing in Medicine*, DOI 10.1007/978-3-319-61924-8_10

for their marketed use. 3D printing is an emerging technology that has brought many new users to the field who may not be familiar with the federal regulations and requirements for medical device clearance or approval. The FDA has a decade of experience with 3D printed medical devices across the industry, the FDA has worked with and provided resources for small businesses developing medical devices. This chapter provides an overview of the overall FDA regulatory framework for medical devices. Discussion topics will include how devices are classified by the agency, premarket regulatory pathways, FDA guidance for specific device types, and resources available to help device developers, users, and clinicians. It will also include a brief summary of FDA's Technical Considerations for Additive Manufacturing of Medical Devices (FDA 2016a). These considerations were published in a Draft Guidance released in May 2016, pending finalization. They are based on internal research performed in the FDA's Office of Science and Engineering Laboratories, with direct input from stakeholders (industry, academia, patient groups) from FDA's first 3D printing workshop held on October 8–9, 2014, and subsequent scientific conferences and public meetings.

10.3 Brief Overview of FDA Regulatory Pathways for Medical Devices

Medical devices span a wide range of products from tongue depressors, to total knee replacements, to implantable cardiac defibrillators, all regulated under the Center for Devices and Radiologic Health (CDRH). A medical device is defined in the Food Drug and Cosmetic Act (FDCA Section 201(h)) as "an instrument, apparatus, implement, machine, contrivance, implant, in vitro reagent, or other similar or related article, including a component part, or accessory which is:

- recognized in the official National Formulary, or the United States Pharmacopoeia, or any supplement to them.
- intended for use in the diagnosis of disease or other conditions, or in the cure, mitigation,

treatment, or prevention of disease, in man or other animals, or
- intended to affect the structure or any function of the body of man or other animals, and which does not achieve its primary intended purposes through chemical action within or on the body of man or other animals and which is not dependent upon being metabolized for the achievement of any of its primary intended purposes."

The FDA evaluates devices using a risk-based framework that outlines the premarket regulatory requirements that a device must satisfy before being marketed in the United States. Several factors in addition to risk help to determine the regulatory classification and evaluation; these include but are not limited to the intended use and indications for use. These two terms are often conflated but they are distinct, as clarified by FDA Guidance, on the 510(k) Program: Evaluating Substantial Equivalence in Premarket Notifications, Section D.1. "Intended use means the general purpose of a device or its function and encompasses the indications for use" (FDA 2014a, b). The more specific term, "indications for use as defined in 21 CFR 814.20(b)(3)(i), describes the disease or condition the device will diagnose, treat, prevent, cure, or mitigate, including a description of the patient population for which the device is intended." Understanding the basic regulatory framework and terminology can be useful for new device developers, engineers, and clinicians.

10.3.1 Resources

Interacting with the FDA may seem like a daunting task, but in fact, 99% of the device manufacturers that contact the FDA are small businesses. Moreover, 74% of those businesses have ten employees or fewer. The medical device industry in particular is a place for small innovative groups to develop new products and technologies. CDRH aims to provide resources to foster that innovation. The FDA website contains a wealth of information for new and experienced medical product developers, manufacturers, sponsors,[1] and consumers. Websites referenced throughout this document will be listed with their hyperlinks in the Additional Online Resources section. Specifically, the CDRH website includes a section called "Device Advice" with comprehensive regulatory information and a series of webinars called "CDRH Learn" that describe FDA practices and regulations. Topics include summary information and how to study and market your device, special topics for specific situations, and postmarket activities. 3D printing has its own set of pages on the FDA site which talk about the types of medical applications for 3D printing as well as providing more details on the FDA's role. More generally, one of the most common ways for FDA to describe policies, interpretations of regulations, and product-specific concerns is through the release of guidance documents, available through a searchable database. CDRH Guidance Documents describe the process and requirements for each type of submission, recommendations for best practices, and specific data that certain device submissions require for thorough evaluation. It is often advantageous to discuss potential devices or medical products with the FDA early in the development or testing process to understand what the FDA will want to see for clearance or approval.

10.3.2 Classification

All medical devices that are currently marketed in the United States are classified by the FDA and can often be used as a guide to determine the regulatory classification of new devices. This information is found in the Code of Federal Regulations (CFR), Title 21, Sections 800–1299 and maintained by the Government Publishing Office website. Searchable information on the classification of marketed medical devices can also be found in the FDA's Product Classification Database. If a device does not fit into one of the existing product classifications (presents a potential new intended use or may raise new questions of safety or effectiveness), its regulatory

classification should be discussed with the FDA. There is an official process, called 513(g), established for sponsors to request a classification of any product if none exists or if the classification is unclear (FDA 2012a, b).

Generally, devices can be divided into three classes. Each class has a specific path to market, requiring a different amount of data. To support submission, there are several ways to formally and informally communicate with the FDA to ask questions about a specific product before it is ready to bring to market (Fig. 10.2).

- Low-risk (Class I) devices which are generally exempt from premarket review.
- Moderate-risk or controlled risk (Class II) devices which typically require review through the Premarket Notification [510(k)] process.
- High-risk or life-sustaining (Class III) devices which typically require review through the premarket approval (PMA) process. Most require clinical study data gathered under an investigational device exemption (IDE).

10.3.2.1 Class I

The vast majority of Class I devices are exempt from the premarket review requirements of Class II and Class III. Instead, these devices need to comply with what are termed general controls that include labeling, manufacturing quality standards, and reporting requirements as well as registration and listing with the FDA (FDA 2014a). One of the principle qualities of a Class I device that is exempt from premarket review is that it presents a very low risk to the patient. However, if a Class I device is being marketed for a new indication for use or employs a fundamentally different technology to achieve the intended use, then it may require a Premarket Notification submission [510(k)] or premarket approval (PMA) based on several factors including the risk that the device may pose to the user or patient.

10.3.2.2 Class II: Premarket Notification [510(k)]

Class II devices include a wide variety of devices that may present moderate risks to patients and users and that do not sustain life. The agency

---

[1]"Sponsor" is the term FDA uses for any person, company, or institution that sends a submission to the FDA.

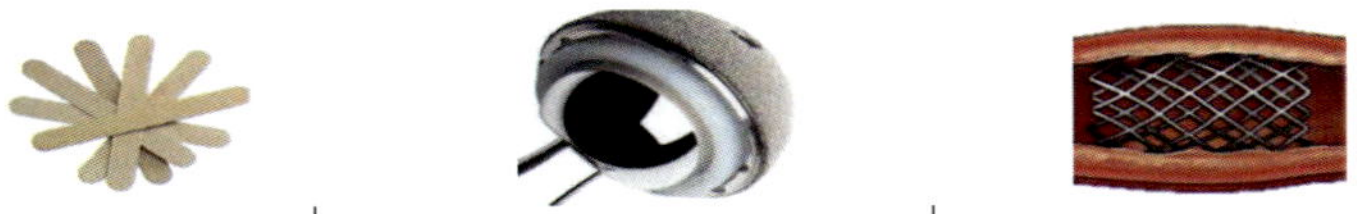

US device class	Class I (exempt)	Class II	Class III
Risk	Low	Moderate	High
Pre-market submission	Registration and listing	510(k)	PMA
Level of evidence	N/A	**Substantial equivalence** to a predicate	**Safety & effectiveness**
Regulatory controls	• General controls	• General controls • Special controls • Devices-specific guidance	• General controls • Device-specific guidance • Manufacturing controls
Post-market Compliance	• Quality System regulations • Some exemptions	• Quality System regulations	• Quality System regulations

Fig. 10.2 The three primary classifications of medical devices used by the FDA and their approximate correlation to European classifications

expects that the risks these devices may present can be mitigated through the use of device-specific special controls. These controls describe the data the FDA needs to effectively evaluate the device as well as best practices for preparing a device for market. They may include but are not limited to preclinical bench testing, animal studies, risk assessment, and suggested labeling. In a minority of cases, clinical data may be required if other data cannot resolve questions of safety and effectiveness brought about by new or different technological characteristics. The majority of Class II devices are required to submit a Premarket Notification [510(k)] for review by the FDA before they can be *cleared* for marketing in the United States (FDA 2014a, b). Sponsors of 510(k) submissions must demonstrate that their submission is *substantially equivalent* to a legally marketed *predicate*, or previously cleared medical device, that has comparable technological characteristics, intended use, and indications for use.

10.3.2.3 Class III: Premarket Approval (PMA)

Devices in the highest-risk classification require premarket approval that demonstrates the safety and effectiveness of the device using all available evidence: preclinical testing, animal studies if applicable, and clinical trials. Risk for Class III

devices may come from a variety of sources, such as their use of novel or untested technologies, materials, or indications for use that make special and general controls insufficient to ensure safety and effectiveness.

10.3.3 Clinical Studies

All clinical studies must be performed with oversight from and approval of an Institutional Review Board (IRB), and significant risk device studies must be approved by the FDA through an investigational device exemption (IDE). Factors that determine if a study poses nonsignificant risk include but are not limited to the type of device, the type of intervention, how much the intervention differs from standard clinical practice, and anticipated adverse events. The FDA is the final arbiter of all clinical study risk determinations. Sponsors may use pre-submission meetings to discuss study protocols, risk determination, endpoints, or other relevant factors that will help collect the correct data to support a PMA or other regulatory submissions. IRB and IDE approvals, as required, must be obtained before enrolling subjects, and IDE submissions should include a report of all previous investigations (e.g., preclinical testing, animal studies) of the device and an investigational plan among other items. See CDRH's Device Advice on IDEs for more information. The CDRH Device Advice website also contains information and guidance on determining if a device is a significant risk and how to apply for an IDE.

The speed of technological development is increasing rapidly and with it, the potential for innovation in medical devices. CDRH has implemented early feasibility studies as a way to "allow for early clinical evaluation of devices to provide proof of principle and initial clinical safety data" (FDA 2013a, b). As with all clinical studies, there must be appropriate benefit-risk analyses and human subject protections. However, unlike traditional IDE studies, early feasibility studies are designed for devices in early development, often before the design has been finalized. The subject enrollment is typically small (ten subjects or less), and the data collected may help gain insight that is not available through preclinical testing or to guide device modifications.

Perspective: Many times, the question is asked, "How do we prove to the FDA that the benefits of the device outweigh the risks and that there is reason to believe the device will be effective?" While the FDA is able to give the final legal approval for a significant risk clinical study to proceed, they are not the target audience for the device (only the submissions). Patients are the beneficiaries and the ones who will be most affected by the device. A more appropriate question might be, "Would a patient who is well informed about the function of the device, the risks of the study, and the potential benefit choose to participate?" The FDA uses benefit-risk analysis (FDA 2012b, 2016d) to make its determinations including the submitted data on the engineering safety, manufacturing controls, potential effectiveness, and patient tolerance for risk (Hunter and Califf 2015) among others. Most devices require understanding a complex mix of medicine, engineering, biology, and other sciences that contribute to the manufacture, use, and function of the device. The FDA staff includes reviewers and scientists from a wide range of disciplines and expertise. In addition, each division has an unmatched knowledge of the history of devices in their area that give them a unique perspective.

10.3.4 Pre-Submission Meetings

Sometimes sponsors may have questions about their device, about the data that FDA may require, or endpoints for their clinical study. Pre-submission meetings (pre-submissions) allow a sponsor to ask specific questions of the agency about their device, study, or aspects of their submission (FDA 2014b). A sponsor can request a pre-submission at any point in the regulatory process including the preclinical testing phase or in response to feedback from FDA about a device submission. Early pre-submissions are especially important for devices using a novel technology or innovation because it gives the agency a glimpse at the device before the marketing (e.g., 510(k), PMA) or IDE submission. When the agency can take time to understand the features and technology in a very novel device, reviewers and scientists are better able to evaluate it and ask appropriate questions to assess safety and effectiveness. This can also benefit sponsors by reducing the number of questions or review rounds needed to come to a final decision.

10.3.5 Other Regulatory Pathways

Premarket notifications [510(k)], premarket approval (PMA), and investigational device exemptions (IDE) are the most common submissions to CDRH for medical devices. There are, however, other pathways that can be used for certain devices.

10.3.5.1 Humanitarian Use Device (HUD)/Humanitarian Device Exemption (HDE)

Some diseases affect small populations, and some specialized treatments are only right for small population within a more prevalent disease. For these cases, the FDA has the HUD/HDE process. Someone who has a potential treatment for one of these small populations can request a Humanitarian Use Device designation for the patient population and indications for use of the device. If the expected patient population is less than 4000 per year (incidence) and other criteria are met, then an HUD may be granted. Other requirements and restrictions are described on the CDRH Device Advice website and in FDA Guidance on Humanitarian Use Device (HUD) Designations (FDA 2013a, b). Once an HUD is granted, the sponsor may submit a Humanitarian Device Exemption (HDE) to allow for the device to be marketed in the United States. In this submission, a sponsor must show that the device is safe and that the probable benefits of the device outweigh the risks, typically with a clinical study.

10.3.5.2 De Novo

Technology is developing at a rapid rate and not all devices with low or moderate risk will have a predicate for a 510(k) submission. To address this, congress and the FDA created a new regulatory submission through the 1997 Food and Drug Administration Modernization Act (FDAMA) (FDA 1997a, b) and the 2012 FDA Safety and Innovation Act (FDASIA) (FDA 2016b). This submission is called for de novo, Latin for "from the beginning" or "newly started." Any person who has a device for which a Class III regulation does not exist and has either "received a determination of Not Substantially Equivalent (NSE) in response to a 510(k) submission" or "who determines there is no legally marketed device upon which to base a determination of substantial equivalence may submit a de novo request." This request reevaluates the automatic Class III designation of the device (FDA 2017). In order to change the classification, data and testing should show that the risk to the patient posed for the de novo device is similar to that of a Class II or Class I device. Likewise, the benefits and risks should be understood well enough to be mitigated through use of general and special controls. Once the reclassification is granted, a de novo device can be used as a predicate to support future 510(k) submissions.

10.3.5.3 Combination Products

Combination products typically use elements of two or more regulated areas such as biologic/device or drug/device to function as a single product. The Code of Federal Regulation defines a combination product more fully (21 CFR 3.2(e)). Some research and development areas such as tissue

engineering frequently yield combination products due to the incorporation of cells within a scaffold or other physical structure. The FDA's Office of Combination Products makes the final determination if a product is a combination product and which regulatory center has the lead review role for that product based on its primary mode of action. Other centers may use different regulatory pathways than those described here.

10.4 Regulatory Landscape for 3D-Printed Medical Devices

10.4.1 Medical Implants and Accessories

Medical device manufacturers were early adopters of 3D printing, but interest in 3D printing medical devices has grown exponentially since 2010. As of 2016, the FDA has over a decade of regulatory experience with 3D-printed products with dozens of cleared medical devices (Fig. 10.3). All of these clearances, approvals, and authorizations have occurred under the existing regulatory framework.

Additive manufacturing is inherently a manufacturing process. The capability to make very complex shapes increase the innovative potential for designers is still only a part of the process of

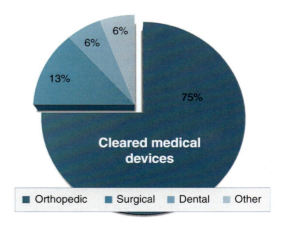

Fig. 10.3 Distribution of 510(k) cleared medical devices using 3D printing by discipline

creating a device. As with any manufacturing process, there are factors that must be considered in the evaluation of safety and effectiveness, but it does not necessarily change the categorization or regulatory classification of a device. In fact, many 3D-printed devices have presented enough evidence to receive 510(k) clearance as substantially equivalent to a more traditionally manufactured device. CDRH is organized into divisions that specialize in certain product areas and have access to expert scientists and clinicians.[2] This specialization allows reviewers to consider devices in their current and historical clinical context. Specialized consultants in areas like 3D printing (additive manufacture) can bring expertise on specific technologies where needed.

10.4.2 Surgical Visualization Models

Software applications for clinical imaging and anatomic visualization are Class II medical devices subject to premarket clearance. The anatomy and data from those applications can be printed to aid visualization, much like a 2D paper printout of an echocardiogram or a 3D print of a heart with congenital defects. The printers and software used to run the printer itself are not typically considered medical devices. If the 3D prints are made for use with a specific device or as a necessary aid to complete a regulated procedure, they may require a regulatory submission (Di Prima et al. 2016). Several large hospitals have set up centers to facilitate printing of surgical models and visualization tools. In addition, multiple material and color prints are being used as training tools to practice different surgical procedures and disease states (Morris 2016; LaFrance 2013; PCHC 2017).

10.4.3 Prosthetics and Quality of Life Accessories

Prosthetics are regulated devices under 21 CFR 890. Many are Class I and exempt from premar-

ket submission, but still benefit from general quality controls. A wide range of prostheses and orthoses are categorized by the regulation, each with its own description and classification. Attachments for prosthetics such as specialty hooks, button pushing devices, or holders for tablets are not typically considered medical devices. Of course, generalizations cannot capture the specific details and differences for every device and intended use. The FDA has final authority to make decisions regarding the classification and regulation of medical devices and provides resources to help sponsors determine where they are in the regulatory framework. Those making prosthetics and these types of devices can search the Device Advice website or Guidance Database for information. They can also contact the Division of Industry and Consumer Education[3] to determine if answering their questions requires a pre-submission meeting.

10.5 Printing Materials

Many types of materials can be additively manufactured, from metals, to polymers, to biological molecules and cells. The intended use, the printing technology, and post-printing steps all factor into the decision of what material to use and what testing to perform.

10.5.1 Characterization

Additive manufacturing builds a part in a way that can melt, sinter, or adhere pieces of material to each other. This can greatly change the physical properties from what is expected from a solid part made from the same material. As always, there are such a variety of medical products that could be made additive manufacturing that it would be impossible to describe the ideal characteristics or specifications for all applications. Most importantly, designers and manufacturers should know as much as they can

---

[2]The CDRH Organizational chart is available on the FDA website.

[3]Contact DICE by email: DICE@fda.hhs.gov or by phone at 1 (800) 638-2041 or (301) 796-7100.

about the 3D printing process they are using. That will form a basis to decide which characteristics of their raw material are essential to achieve consistent results. For instance, in powder bed fusion systems, the size and shape of the powder is extremely important for achieving even spreading across the powder bed and consistent melting when energy is applied. Similarly, the powder may change over time as it is used, so the number of reuses and the mixture of new and used powder can be very influential on the final product properties. Equally important are environmental effects such as humidity, exposure to light and heat, or material age. These types of questions are not unique to powder bed fusion systems. All types of printing materials will have their unique set of features that will change with printing method, time, or application and must be characterized. Achieving consistency is one of the primary goals of a manufacturing quality system. There are different techniques to fully assess a manufacturing process including a Process Failure Mode and Effects Analysis (PFMEA). A PFMEA can assist in systematically identifying possible points of failure or variability in a system and then determining the appropriate mitigation strategies to use based on the risk of each failure mode. See the Engineering Tools section for more details.

It may seem like materials that are already used in medical products such as titanium alloy (Ti6Al4V) would be the same for subtractive and additive manufacturing. In fact, in this particular case, the heat of the powder bed melting process can preferentially volatilize aluminum (Mukherjee et al. 2016) and change the composition of the final alloy. Characterization of material properties, including its chemistry, is especially important for polymers and biologically derived molecules where many parameters can be affected by the printing process. Some material components such as residual monomers, additives, or contaminants may adversely affect tissues if they are not appropriately handled during processing or removed from the final part. Characterizing the raw materials and the process steps can help elucidate where undesirable variability or contaminants may occur, and it may facilitate implementation of mitigation strategies.

10.5.2 Biological Suitability

Some 3D printing materials are almost identical to materials used in other types of manufacturing, while others have been developed especially for 3D printing. However, just like other forms of manufacturing, this does not mean that all printable materials will be suitable for use in medical products. Materials should be matched to their intended use for physical, chemical, and biological properties. There is a common misconception that FDA clears materials for specific medical uses. This is typically not the case. CDRH evaluates the materials used in a device in the context of the device and its intended use.

For example, total joint replacements are often made from titanium alloy (Ti6Al4V) which has been used very frequently. Overall, it is considered to be biocompatible for this use. However, Ti6Al4V has not been approved for brain aneurysm clips because the aluminum in the alloy can specifically be toxic to brain cells. In this case, titanium alloy would not be very biocompatible for this use. The longer clinical history a material has in a specific device area, the more data and experience is available to show the safety and effectiveness of that material. Sometimes new materials are developed for a particular application like joint implants, new data emerges about existing materials like titanium alloy, or new features and technologies are integrated into previous designs. The new information can then be incorporated into future evaluations of the material.

Once a material set of possible materials are chosen for a particular application, they can be tested for adverse biological effects using the International Standard ISO 10993 "Biological Evaluation of Medical Devices." In June 2016, the FDA finalized guidance on the use of the standard (FDA 2016c). It has 20 parts that each focus on a different aspect of biocompatibility testing, applicable to a very wide range of materials and applications. The FDA publishes information on its website about the general application of standards and other guidance documents that may have device-specific requirements or recommendations. Among other factors, the duration of contact with the body and the risk posed by the device will influence the type and rigor of testing that is needed to show biocompatibility.

Some information on raw materials may contain the words "medical grade" or terms related to medical use. This is not an indication that the material is FDA approved or cleared. Rather, it may mean the manufacturer has subjected the material to ISO-10993 standard tests or the older USP Class 6 testing. Material suppliers should be able to provide all test results on their products and the lab(s) where they were tested through their website or upon request. Third-party testing by a recognized independent lab is one of the best ways to ensure that the results will be consistent for a product and comparable across different products. Sometimes an assessment of patient exposure to a material coupled with the existing testing is enough to show that the material is biocompatible for a specific application. Materials that have been used in previously cleared or approved medical devices often have a master file with the FDA (FDA 2002). This file gives the FDA confidential access to proprietary information that the material supplier may not wish to share publicly or with customers. It is a mechanism to protect intellectual property and ensure the FDA has enough information to evaluate a product. Many material specifications and tests may be stored in the master file. However, as described, there are many elements to these standards, and the material supplier may not have completed exhaustive testing. The printing process or other production steps may also modify the material through additives, physical exposure, or chemical treatment, thereby altering the biocompatibility profile and necessitating additional testing.

Material characteristics of the raw material, including biocompatibility, are important, but a medical product functions and is evaluated based on the final finished device. That means that each step of the product workflow must be taken into account when evaluating the suitability of a material, and the final device itself will often be the subject of many of the performance and safety tests.

10.6 The Design Process

Medical devices cover such a wide range of technologies that it is nearly impossible to describe all the workflows, design processes, and manufacturing controls in one place. Each step in design and manufacturing processes are interdependent on the others, and sometimes it is not easy to determine what variables or steps are most critical to quality. Frameworks such as a Process Failure Mode and Effects Analysis and user-centric design help evaluate processes in a methodical way. The FDA published guidance specifically on structuring the design processes to practically implement quality assurance (FDA 1997a, b).

Modern software packages can easily make intricate features such as lattice structures, porous coatings, and patient-specific designs, but it is up to the designer, sometimes collaborating with a clinical team, to determine if those structures and features meet performance and safety specifications. By considering best practices, documentation, and clinical use throughout the entire research and development process, designers can identify hurdles early, make iterative improvements, and even help navigate the regulatory process.

10.6.1 Engineering Tools

There are several engineering methodologies that can help designers develop products that anticipate possible risk factors, build in mitigations, and ensure that features critical to the quality of the device are adequately controlled. These processes can be used for the design of the device, evaluating steps in the printing process and even assessing the interactions between users/patients and device or part. Some examples of those tools are described below.

10.6.1.1 Failure Mode Effects Analysis (FMEA)

The Quality Toolbox (Tague 2005) defines FMEA as a step-by-step approach for identifying all possible failures in a design, manufacturing, or assembly process or product. Importantly, this method requires an interdisciplinary team that understands all aspects of the product from design to end use, including the end users. A large table is assembled with one failure mode on each line. Once identified, the risk posed by that failure, the probability of it occurring, and possible mitigation strategies are listed on that row (Table 10.1).

10.6.1.2 User-Centric and Patient-Centric Design

Intuitive or user-friendly designs are increasingly used in modern technology and applications, but device designers are often not clinicians or patients. Knowing exactly how a device is used in the real world by clinicians and how it will affect the patient is an important part of ensuring the device is both safe and effective. FDA's Guidance on "Applying Human Factors and Usability Engineering to Medical Devices" outlines generally how to apply these principles for regulated products (FDA 2016d). In addition, The U.S. Department of Health and Human Services maintains usability.gov, which provides tools, surveys, and best practices for how to perform user preference and performance. In these contexts, there can be many types of users, for example, the image processing personnel, part designers, printer operators, clinicians, and patients. Going through these exercises can bring out small tweaks that may make a process more streamlined, instructions clearer, device features more comfortable, or even adapt visual features to bring attention to a particular function at an appropriate time.

10.6.2 Patient-Matching Workflow

Making a device patient-matched entails applying a set of steps or changes to a design that will yield products with the very similar performance and safety profiles, but that fit a specific patient's anatomy or physiology. The quality of patient imaging can be especially important for these devices because standard clinical CT or MRI scans may or may not provide enough resolution or contrast to define essential anatomic features to perform patient matching. This is again a situation where fully understanding the process and the design needs can help determine the correct strategies, whether that is using a different imaging method or defining stricter imaging protocols. Once the image volume is captured and the anatomy is isolated or segmented, the patient-specific design features can be placed. This may involve interactions with a clinical team in a local or remote location. As designs are iterated it is important to track design versions and maintain patient privacy according to Health Insurance Portability and Accountability Act (HIPAA) regulations (DHHS 2005). Documentation and identifying marks may help prevent an old version of a file being printed for a patient or the wrong patient's device being sent.

10.7 The Manufacturing Process

10.7.1 Software/Hardware Interactions

Every software and embedded firmware has its own quirks and idiosyncrasies. Many groups across many industries "freeze" software and hardware updates after validating particularly complex processes. This ensures that there will not be any unexpected changes or errors in outputs caused simply by updating versions. Even changing something as simple as the smoothing algorithm used to generate files can alter outputs depending on the type of device and features it contains. Maintaining a set of test coupons or other parts that represent the edges of the design envelope can facilitate reevaluation of the software workflow.

Most printer types build each layer in a rostered (like an old television screen) or linear fashion where a single point of energy or material delivery is moved across that layer of the build volume. This build path takes time to traverse an entire layer and can affect the way

Table 10.1 Example FMEA for a button function

Potential failure mode	Potential effect of the failure	Potential cause of failure	Severity	Probability	Probability of detection during production	Risk priority	Current prevention strategy	Current detection method	Recommended actions	Adjusted risk
Power stays on after pressing "off"	Battery drains	Button is too difficult to press	Moderate	Very low	High	Low	Use tactile feedback levels from HE75	Design control on button pressure	None	As low as possible
		Power short from improper insulation	Moderate	Moderate	Moderate	Moderate	Rubber buttons	Product sampling	Add gasket to reduce likelihood of moisture infiltration	Low

The risk priority is a combination of severity of the harm, probability of occurrence, and probability of detection. The goal of an FMEA is to reduce product failures and associated risks to an acceptable level each part is made, for example, the cooling time between when an outer layer and adjacent layer can affect their adhesion. Likewise, if a contour is always started and stopped at the same location, there may be a seam in the part that can affect the mechanical properties of the final part. For printing that involves cells, this can be even more important as time can be limited. Control of the build path is sometimes embedded within the printer and sometimes is handled by third-party software. In either case, having an understanding of what is happening while each layer is being built can help troubleshoot problems and facilitate consistent results.

10.7.2 Building a Part

Many of the unique aspects of additive manufacturing arise when preparing a part to be built. It is important to understand the limits of a printer before using it for production because each printer may require slightly different settings to make acceptable parts based on the material, hardware, local environment, or other factors. For all printer types and models, there are several important factors that can help achieve consistent results. The following sections describe some of these factors that may not always be in the forefront when planning or assessing build processes. Each printer and process will have a unique set of steps or parameters that are critical to quality (CTQ) for the intended use.

10.7.2.1   Part Orientation and Location in the Build Volume

One of the most obvious differences between additive manufacturing and other types of manufacturing is that mechanical strength and structural integrity between layers (in the z direction) is typically lower than within a layer. Therefore, the orientation of a print becomes an important factor in determining if it meets specifications. In addition, the proximity of parts in the print space can also adversely affect performance by allowing energy delivered to one part to be absorbed by another part, and the management

of orientation and heat distribution is critical to the accuracy of devices in metal additive manufacturing.

10.7.2.2   Support Materials

Many printing processes require support materials to be added so that the layers of material can be built up without collapsing. These supports must then be removed after printing to obtain the final part. Too few supports can lead to unstable or poorly fused sections of material, whereas too many supports can make removal and surface finishing more difficult. Whether automated or manual algorithms are used to place these supports, they can affect the surface finish and performance of the final part. Careful consideration of the remove method (physical or chemical) can help prevent residues of the removal process being left on the part.

10.7.2.3   Machine Parameters

The printers themselves also have software or firmware that can affect the way a part is built. Parameters such as set temperatures, dwell times, and print speed may all be controlled and monitored by the machine itself. The variability allowed in these parameters could affect the consistency of the build process. In addition, the aforementioned build path may be set in the machine as well (e.g., rotating the start coordinate with every layer or drawing the outer contours before the inner fill). The machine parameters necessary to keep build quality consistent can also be affected by input parameters that have to be monitored and controlled separately. For instance, the ambient environment (e.g., humidity, temperature) of the printer may have a great effect on the materials. Likewise, the raw material characteristics discussed in the previous section can change, also affect the machine performance.

10.7.2.4   Post-Processing

Almost all parts made with additive manufacturing will require some type of post-processing. This may be support removal, heat treatment, cleaning, sterilization, or a variety of other machining tasks to make the part take its final shape. Each of these steps can have effects on the residual stress in the part, surface finish, or residues. Geometric, mechanical, and biological characterization of any part after all post-processing steps are completed will ensure that those effects are taken into account. For specific tests in specific circumstances, there may be no additional benefit to performing it after all post-processing, and those can be evaluated on a case-by-case basis to make the process more efficient.

10.8 Verification and Process Validation

Two key principles that undergird any quality system are verification and validation. Verification is the measurement of a feature or property to assess whether or not it falls within a specified nominal range or tolerance. If every part is checked for that feature, it is said to be fully verified. Some properties cannot be checked without damaging or destroying a part such as mechanical strength or fatigue life. In that case the system must be validated. Validation would occur on the production equipment using the final production process. Inputs such as environmental conditions, raw material characteristics, operating parameters, etc. are all monitored closely, and each product is then tested (verified) to evaluate all the necessary specifications. Once a process is validated, it means that if the input criteria are within a defined range, then the output product will meet nominal specifications and does not have to be fully verified. Validation is reevaluated through statistical sampling or other testing methods.

Validation becomes especially important in additively manufacturing where there are many variables that can affect the final outcome, some of which are not currently possible to measure. In addition, patient-specific devices may all be slightly different so verification can be more difficult or impossible. In these cases, it is important to think about validation even in the design stage where you are defining the "design envelope" and determining the workflow that will ensure patient-specific devices meet performance goals.

10.8.1 Quality Systems

The FDA has developed a comprehensive set of quality system regulations and guidance documents to help small and large businesses develop and maintain good manufacturing practices for medical devices. These can help to ensure that medical devices are continually produced to meet specifications time after time. The techniques are most often used in manufacturing settings, but they can also be used by researchers or clinicians who are developing techniques and products that may later be commercialized. The quality system regulations are made to be flexible so they apply to almost any device and as many manufacturing scenarios as possible (Tartal 2014).

10.8.2 Monitoring

Since every part made by a validated process is not completely characterized (verified), monitoring the system becomes an important part of ensuring the quality of each part. Typically, samples are taken from a manufactured group of parts (lot). Those parts are then subjected to a full battery of destructive and non-destructive testing. CDHR Additive Manufacturing (AM) Working Group makes it more difficult to determine how many parts constitute a lot, and in the case of patient-specific parts, there may only be one. Other methods can be used to still control the build quality over time. These may include checks on the raw materials, environmental monitoring, in-process monitoring (e.g., temperature at energy delivery point, machine status), and use of test coupons.

10.8.3 Test Coupons

Test coupons are pieces that represent a certain feature or features of the final part and are made in a way that replicates a worst-case scenario for the final finished part. During validation, worst-case locations and orientations in the build volume are identified; test coupons can then be built at these locations and evaluated for various performance criteria. If the test coupons are representative of the final part and they meet performance specifications at the worst-case build locations, it can increase confidence that parts made during the same build will also meet specification. It can be difficult to determine what makes a test coupon "representative" depending on the complexity of the part being produced. There may also be more than one worst-case or "representative" test coupon based on the tests being performed.

10.9   Conclusions

3D printing is a process, like any other manufacturing process; the wide range of technologies available and the freedoms imparted may bring many factors into the fore. Designers and manufacturers will continue to build their comfort levels with their processes by following best practices, quality systems, and other good manufacturing frameworks. Whether the end goal is to market a product, perform research, or develop new technologies, the best practices published by the FDA, embodied in standards, and implemented through engineering tools can be useful for any person or group—no matter how small. In the end, the risk profile of each product and process will dictate what measures must be taken to ensure that the final products meet specifications time after time. Considering quality control and quality system processes early in the development process, even at the laboratory research phases, can both help translation of product ideas into commercial products and can also foster innovation through improved process understanding.

FDA and CDRH both have innovation teams and websites that can provide early assistance for emerging technologies and to nontraditional innovators. The FDA continues to build a knowledge base for 3D printing and other emerging technologies through internal research, participating in standards like the ASTM F42 Additive Manufacturing Standards Committee and public-private partnerships such as America Makes. FDA personnel also attend academic, clinical, industry, and user conferences (such as the Orthopedic Research Society Annual Meeting, Radiological Society of North America Annual Meeting, and Special Interest Group Meetings, Society for Manufacturing Engineers' RAPID, and Additive Manufacturing Users Group) to relate and learn best practices across the industry. Increased access to information and communication has been one of the major topics during industry meetings, and in some ways it has also been one of the strengths of the 3D printing community. Gaining insight from FDA's website and publications, and contacting the FDA early in your design or development process can help streamline submission logistics, experimental design, and trial design. The FDA is working to foster innovation through 3D printing while maintaining the high quality of safe and effective medical devices that patients and clinicians have come to expect.

Additional Online Resources
- 3D Printing of Medical Devices: http://www.fda.gov/3dprinting
- CDRH Device Advice: http://www.fda.gov/MedicalDevices/DeviceRegulationandGuidance
- CDRH Device Advice- Investigational Device Exemption (IDE): http://www.fda.gov/MedicalDevices/DeviceRegulationandGuidance/HowtoMarketYourDevice/InvestigationalDeviceExemptionIDE
- CDRH Innovation Team: http://www.fda.gov/AboutFDA/CentersOffices/OfficeofMedicalProductsandTobacco/CDRH/CDRHInnovation/
- CDRH Learn: http://www.fda.gov/training/cdrhlearn
- CDRH Offices and Organization: https://www.fda.gov/AboutFDA/CentersOffices/OfficeofMedicalProductsandTobacco/CDRH/CDRHOffices
- Electronic Code of Federal Regualtions: http://www.ecfr.gov/
- FDA Innovation Team: https://www.fda.gov/AboutFDA/Innovation
- Guidance Documents Database: http://www.fda.gov/RegulatoryInformation/Guidances
- Product Classification Database (Medical Devices): http://www.accessdata.fda.gov/scripts/cdrh/cfdocs/cfpcd/classification.cfm

Acknowledgments We would like to thank Matthew Di Prima, Jennifer Kelly, David Hwang, and Laura Ricles of the CDRH Additive Manufacturing Working Group for their help in compiling this information and their continuing efforts in 3D printing regulation, research, and public education.

References

Association for the Advancement of Medical Instrumnetation (AAMI), FDA focus on postmarket benefit–risk for medical devices. 2016. Available from: http://www.aami.org/productspublications/articledetail.aspx?ItemNumber=3707. Cited 4 Aug 2016.

Di Prima M, et al. Additively manufactured medical products – the FDA perspective. 3D Print Med. 2016;2(1)

FDA/CDRH. Food and Drug Administration Modernization Act (FDAMA) of 1997a. Available from: http://www.fda.gov/RegulatoryInformation/Legislation/SignificantAmendmentstotheFDCAct/FDAMA/.

FDA/CDRH. Design control guidance for medical device manufacturers. 1997b. Available from: http://www.fda.gov/downloads/MedicalDevices/.../ucm070642.pdf. 11 Mar 1997

FDA/CDRH. Medical device premarket approval: master files. 2002. Available from: http://www.fda.gov/MedicalDevices/DeviceRegulationandGuidance/HowtoMarketYourDevice/PremarketSubmissions/PremarketApprovalPMA/ucm142714.htm.

FDA/CDRH. FDA and industry procedures for section 513(g) requests for information under the federal food, drug, and cosmetic act. 2012a. Available from: http://www.fda.gov/downloads/MedicalDevices/DeviceRegulationandGuidance/GuidanceDocuments/UCM209851.pdf. 6 Apr 2012.

FDA/CDRH. Factors to consider when making benefit-risk determinations in medical device premarket approvals and de novo classifications. 2012b. Available from: http://www.fda.gov/MedicalDevices/DeviceRegulationandGuidance/GuidanceDocuments/ucm267829.htm. 28 Mar 2012.

FDA/CDRH. Investigational device exemptions (IDEs) for Early feasibility medical device clinical studies, including certain first in human (FIH) studies. 2013a. Available from: http://www.fda.gov/downloads/medicaldevices/deviceregulationandguidance/guidancedocuments/ucm279103.pdf. 1 Oct 2013.

FDA/CDRH. Humanitarian Use Device (HUD) Designations. 2013b. Available from: https://www.fda.gov/downloads/ForIndustry/DevelopingProductsforRareDiseasesConditions/DesignatingHumanitarianUseDevicesHUDS/LegislationRelatingtoHUDsHDEs/UCM336515.pdf. 24 Jan 2013.

FDA/CDRH. Evaluating substantial equivalence in premarket notifications [510(k)]. 2014a. Available from: http://www.fda.gov/downloads/MedicalDevices/.../UCM284443.pdf. 28 Jul 2014.

FDA/CDRH. Requests for feedback on medical device submissions: the pre-submission program and meetings with Food and Drug Administration staff. Available from: http://www.fda.gov/downloads/medicaldevices/deviceregulationandguidance/guidancedocuments/ucm311176.pdf. 18 Feb 2014b.

FDA/CDRH. Technical considerations for additive manufactured devices. 2016a. Available from: https://www.fda.gov/ucm/groups/fdagov-public/@fdagov-meddevgen/documents/document/ucm499809.pdf 10 May 2016.

FDA/CDRH. Food and Drug Administration Safety and Innovation Act (FDASIA). 2016b. Available from: http://www.fda.gov/RegulatoryInformation/Legislation/SignificantAmendmentstotheFDCAct/FDASIA/ucm20027187.htm.

FDA/CDRH. Use of International Standard ISO 10993–1, Biological evaluation of medical devices – Part 1: Evaluation and testing within a risk management process. 2016c. Available from: http://www.fda.gov/downloads/medicaldevices/deviceregulationandguidance/guidancedocuments/ucm348890.pdf. 16 June 2016.

FDA/CDRH. Applying human factors and usability engineering to medical devices 2016d. https://www.fda.gov/downloads/MedicalDevices/.../UCM259760.pdf 3 Feb 2016.

FDA/CDRH. Evaluation of automatic class III designation (de novo) summaries. 2017. Available from: http://www.fda.gov/AboutFDA/CentersOffices/OfficeofMedicalProductsandTobacco/CDRH/CDRHTransparency/ucm232269.htm.

Hunter NL, Califf RM. FDA's patient preference initiative: the need for evolving tools and policies, in FDA voice. 2015. September 25, 2015. Available from: https://blogs.fda.gov/fdavoice/index.php/tag/patient-preference-initiative.

LaFrance A. To help solve challenging cardiac problems, doctors at Children's press 'print'. The Washington Post. 2013.

Morris J. Q&A: How Mayo is integrating 3D printing into the operating room. In: Schaust S, editor. Twin cities business. 2016. http://tcbmag.com/News/Recent-News/2016/April/Q-A-How-Mayo-Is-Integrating-3D-Printing-Into-The-O.

Mukherjee T, et al. Printability of alloys for additive manufacturing. Sci Rep. 2016;6:19717.

Phoenix Children's Heart Center. Cardiac 3D print lab. Available from: http://heart.phoenixchildrens.org/cardiac-3d-print-lab. 2017.

Tague NR. The quality toolbox, vol. 2. Milwaukee: ASQ Quality Press; 2005. p. 584.

Tartal J. Quality system regulation overview. FDA Small Business Regulatory Education for Industry (REdI). 2014. Available from: http://www.fda.gov/downloads/Drugs/DevelopmentApprovalProcess/SmallBusinessAssistance/UCM408002.pdf. 17 June 2014.

US Department of Health and Human Services. The HIPAA privacy rule. 2005. Available from: http://www.hhs.gov/hipaa/for-professionals/privacy/.

Quality and Safety of 3D-Printed Medical Models

11

Dimitrios Mitsouras, Elizabeth George, and Frank J. Rybicki

Two related advancements are among the necessary requirements for 3D printing to more completely realize its potential for clinical care: the first is that models are reimbursed. The second is that a complete quality and safety program must be developed. This chapter will highlight advances that the field has made collectively, and it will also point out the deficiencies that should be viewed as "action items" for current and emerging leaders in the field to tackle. In some ways, 3D printing can be considered as a new method to display data, following the progression in technology that the picture archiving and communication system (PACS) made over the film alternator, and then to supplement that data with strategies to enhance care pathways. Regardless of how the field is considered, we believe that a very useful strategy to envision the work to be done is to follow the steps necessary to propel this new technology to wider use in patient care.

Recently, the Radiological Society of North America (RSNA) launched the Special Interest Group for 3D Printing, emphasizing the importance of 3D printing in medicine and providing an organizational infrastructure. The Guidelines Subcommittee of the RSNA Special Interest Group, led by Dr. Adnan Sheikh of the University of Ottawa, is actively working to establish recommendations that will represent important practice parameters. This includes both the conversion of DICOM images to Standard Tessellation Language (STL) files and the design of nonanatomic STL files (e.g., surgical guides) based on anatomy visualized in DICOM images and the subsequent 3D printing of models from those files.

One important pathway toward general acceptance, and ultimately reimbursement, for 3D printing among specific clinical scenarios, is the development of guidelines akin to those in place American College of Radiology (ACR) (Appropriateness Criteria® (AC). The RSNA Special Interest Group is formulating an algorithm to start, using well-established clinical scenarios. The usual three categories of appropriateness, as adopted by the AC, can be divided into usually appropriate, maybe appropriate, and rarely appropriate, and in general these have become integrated to clinical decision support engines. The role for appropriateness in 3D printing is critically important since the assessment

D. Mitsouras, Ph.D. (✉)
Applied Imaging Science Lab, Department of Radiology, Brigham and Women's Hospital, 75 Francis St, Boston, MA 02115, USA

Faculty of Medicine, Department of Biochemistry Microbiology and Immunology, The University of Ottawa, Ottawa, ON, Canada
e-mail: dmitsouras@alum.mit.edu

E. George, M.D.
Department of Radiology, Brigham and Women's Hospital, Boston, MA, USA
e-mail: egeorge6@partners.org

F.J. Rybicki, M.D., Ph.D.
Department of Radiology, The University of Ottawa Faculty of Medicine and The Ottawa Hospital Research Institute, Ottawa, ON, Canada
e-mail: frybicki@toh.ca

© Springer International Publishing AG 2017
F.J. Rybicki, G.T. Grant (eds.), *3D Printing in Medicine*, DOI 10.1007/978-3-319-61924-8_11

for each of the clinical indications can be vetted among multidisciplinary groups, and the format of appropriateness enables organization of the literature.

Next to practice parameters and Appropriateness Criteria, the ACR model addresses quality control (QC) of a technology used for medical imaging. For 3D printing used to assist anatomic visualization, we believe QC will revolve around ensuring accuracy and reproducibility. At present, a printer producing anatomic models used for visualizing anatomy is viewed as equivalent to a film printer, making copies—albeit three-dimensional—of DICOM images, and thus is not regulated by the Food and Drug Administration (FDA) (Di Prima et al. 2016). However, this view may change in the future (Christensen and Rybicki 2017). It is however noted that 3D printer considerations are, and will remain, within the FDA purview when a printer is used in the process of manufacturing medical devices (FDA 2016).

Independent of the future landscape of FDA regulation, it is important to document the quality and safety of physical models produced by a 3D printer so that they can be most effective for their intended use. The ACR defines QC as "distinct technical procedures that ensure the production of a satisfactory product (i.e., high-quality diagnostic images)" (ACR 2012, 2015). These procedures are implemented primarily via the use of resolution and contrast phantoms to test imaging system fidelity. Similar to these QC testing guidelines, we believe that quality control testing of 3D printers will involve the use of specific phantoms that are to be regularly printed in order to ensure the production of a satisfactory product, in this case high-quality medical models. Much work in this arena, reviewed below, is currently underway to design and validate such phantoms specifically for use in clinical 3D printing. Whenever a digital reference standard of the intended medical model is available, mathematical metrics can also be used to establish procedures to determine the overall accuracy of a 3D-printed model. More importantly, such mathematical measures of accuracy can be used to develop interpretive quality assurance processes for radiologists and technologists involved in the creation of 3D-printed models

(George et al. 2017). This is an active area of research in our group and elsewhere, and advances in this developing arena are also reviewed below. A final procedure that can be used for medical 3D printing QC is surgical or pathological correlation (Weinstock et al. 2015); this is also included in the ACR QC procedures (ACR 2012, 2015). This is straightforward for anatomic models that are 3D-printed for surgical planning or intraoperative navigation. Measurements made on the printed models can be directly compared to those made on the surgically exposed tissues (George et al. 2017; Gelaude et al. 2008) or on cadaveric specimens, a proviso that the source DICOM images used to generate the 3D printed model were acquired with the tissue in situ (George et al. 2017; Gelaude et al. 2008), to ensure that the segmentation and processing procedures are identical to those that would be used for in vivo images. Below, we describe techniques and advances for each of these QC procedures.

11.1 Phantom-Based Quality Control

In the context of 3D printing equipment, quality control is likely to rely on printer dimensional accuracy. As discussed in Chap. 2, 3D printer resolutions are typically significantly higher (<0.3 mm in all three axes) than those of most clinical imaging modalities. Resolution is the smallest scale that a 3D printer can reproduce and is only one factor affecting accuracy. Accuracy instead refers to the degree of agreement between the dimensions of the printed object compared to those intended, that is, the dimensions of the digital object stored in a STL or AMF file (Braian et al. 2016).

A number of meticulous studies using both geometric phantoms and anatomic models have reported that dimensional errors with most 3D printing modalities are <1 mm and, with current professional hardware, typically <0.5 mm (Table 11.1) (George et al. 2017). For most medical applications, this level of inaccuracy can be considered negligible. Furthermore, 3D printers have high reproducibility, as is expected since the

Table 11.1 Studies reporting 3D printer accuracy by comparison of design STL versus printed model dimensions using commercial 3D printing equipment (>$5000)

Tested geometry	Printing technology	Absolute difference; mean ± SD (range) [mm, unless otherwise noted]	Relative difference; mean ± SD (range) [%]
Skull and mandible (El-Katatny et al. 2010)	Professional FDM	0.1 ± 0.1 (0.0–0.2)	0.2 ± 0.2% (0.0–0.6%)
Skull and mandible (Salmi et al. 2013)	SLS, polyamide	0.9 ± 0.4 (max: 1.9)	0.8 ± 0.3% (max: 1.4%)
	Binder jet	0.8 ± 0.53 (max: 1.7)	0.7 ± 0.4% (max: 1.6%)
	Material jet	0.2 ± 0.1 (max: 0.5)	0.2 ± 0.1% (max: 0.5%)
Geometric models defined in ISO 12836 for dental restoration (Braian et al. 2016)	SLS, polyamide	Dimensions: 0.06 ± 0.06 (0–0.2) Angles: 0.56 ± 0.47° (0.07°–1.23°)	Dimensions: 0.9 ± 1.2% (0.0–4.1%) Angles: 3.4 ± 2.73% (0.4–7.2%)
	Material jet (equipment A)	Dimensions: 0.02 ± 0.04 (0.0–0.18) Angles: 0.34 ± 0.24° (0.08°–0.64°)	Dimensions: 0.2 ± 0.1% (0.0–0.4%) Angles: 2.0 ± 1.4% (0.5–3.7%)
	Material jet (equipment B)	Dimensions: 0.04 ± 0.03 (0–0.09) Angles: 0.53 ± 0.37° (0.23°–1.05°)	Dimensions: 0.5 ± 0.4% (0–1.39%) Angles: 3.2 ± 2.1% (1.4–6%)
Complex geometric model (Teeter et al. 2015)	SLS, stainless steel	0.01 ± 0.02 (0–0.09)[a]	1.5 ± 3.2% (0–17.8%)[a]

Abbreviations: *SLS* selective laser sintering; *FDM* fused deposition material
[a]Excluding features <0.3 mm

components of well-calibrated, non-failing equipment tend to function nearly identically across runs. One study using SLA, for example, found the reproducibility of printing a skull model to be better than 0.07 mm in all three dimensions across seven prints (George et al. 2017).

Specific technical procedures that implement the basic methodology developed in these phantom-based studies have already been described in the medical literature toward establishing an in-hospital clinical 3D printer QC program (Matsumoto et al. 2015; Leng et al. 2017; Wake et al. 2017). In these procedures, QC phantoms containing features of sizes and shapes relevant for medical 3D printing have been digitally designed with precisely known dimensions in a computer-aided design (CAD) program. These digital QC models can be printed either at regular intervals (for preventive maintenance) or along with every patient model. Physical measurements of the printed QC phantom are then compared with the (design) dimensions of the digital model (Matsumoto et al. 2015; Wake et al. 2017). The

first QC phantom proposed for medical 3D printing (Matsumoto et al. 2015; Leng et al. 2017) contained 0.5–2 linear pair resolution bars per mm (Fig. 11.1). "Second-generation" phantoms have been developed to address more complex shapes, including spherical, cylindrical, hexagonal, conical, and spiral features, both extruding and negative-shaped (i.e., holes of the prescribed shape) (Leng et al. 2017). Whenever possible, manual Vernier caliper measurements should be replaced by more precise and more numerous dimensional measurements of the printed phantoms, for example, via the use of 3D laser scanning or CNC coordinate measuring machines (Liacouras 2017).

Recently, QC phantoms composed of two components that contain mirror features (i.e., positive and corresponding negative) have been proposed (Leng et al. 2017). Such phantoms enable a fit test to be used instead of physical measurements (Leng et al. 2017), simply inserting the positive half of the phantom (with features extruding) into the negative side of the phantom (with the corresponding depressions).

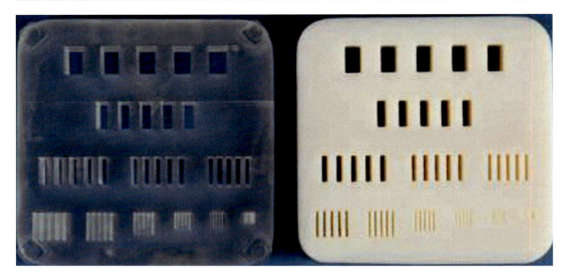

Fig. 11.1 Example of phantom for implementing 3D printing equipment quality control procedures developed at the Mayo Clinic. Reproduced with Permission from Leng S et al., 3D Printing in Medicine, 2017:in press

A successful fit with no visible gaps would presumably attest to printer accuracy. This approach should not be used without some physical measurements, as phantoms printed with an incorrect scaling factor will still pass a fit test. An alternative we propose is to have one half of the fit test QC phantom manufactured using legacy manufacturing (e.g., injection molding, computer numerically controlled [CNC] milling, or laser cutting) and printing the other half with the 3D printer. A successful fit of these two halves would additionally confirm dimensional accuracy of the printed model.

It is important that QC phantoms for medical 3D printing contain features that extend in all three axes and that they also include overhangs that extend in all three axes, as different printer technologies have different accuracy characteristics for such features (George et al. 2017; Pang et al. 1995; Teeter et al. 2015). Furthermore, QC phantoms should ideally be printed using the same materials as the specific medical application for which quality control is being performed (Wake et al. 2017; Teeter et al. 2015), including color (Wake et al. 2017) as this may be achieved using different material chemistries.

11.2 Mathematical Metrics of Quality Control

Comparing agreement between two models of a tissue is a second approach toward establishing quality and safety of medical 3D printing. The two models can be two STL models, each derived from a different segmentation of a tissue depicted in a single DICOM image data set, for example each segmentation performed by a different radiologist. This scenario is useful for quality assurance (QA). The two STL files can also be the initially designed STL to be printed, and a digitized version of the printed model. This scenario is useful for QC of the individual print. A printed model can be digitized, for example, using 3D laser scanning, or tomographic imaging such as CT, and potentially even MRI (George et al. 2017; Mitsouras et al. 2017). Optical scanners are preferred as they have much higher precision (<0.01 mm) compared to CT and MRI, but they are limited to only assessing the outer surface of a model. Once the two STL models to compare are obtained there are two mathematical procedures that can be used to perform such comparisons.

11.2.1 Model Surface Distances

The first approach is to compare the "distance" between STL models. Conceptually, there is a minimum distance from an arbitrary point located on one STL surface to the other STL surface. This distance can be computed for any number of representative points (typically the nodes of the triangular STL mesh), thereby yielding a distribution of distances that pos-sesses an average and standard deviation that together convey a quantitative assessment of the overall difference between the two models (Fig. 11.2).

This approach provides a simple comparison between STL models (George et al. 2017; Leng et al. 2017; Mitsouras et al. 2017) that can be used for QC of individual printed models. Individual printed model QC is necessary since an anatomic model may fail to print in a given

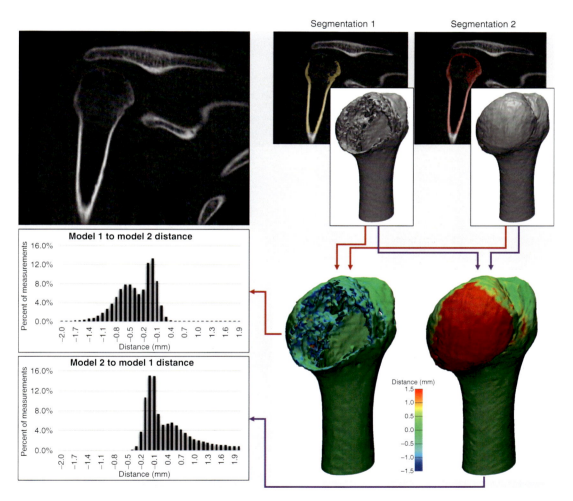

Fig. 11.2 Humerus segmented from CT by two different operators; segmentation 1 was fully automated (bone 226 Hounsfield Unit threshold), while segmentation 2 was manually edited. The former model is missing a portion of the humeral head. Comparing the two models using an STL distance metric to quantitatively assess model agreement is not meaningful; the mean distance from model 1 to model 2 is -0.36 ± 0.43 mm (range, -2.72–2.22 mm), while that from model 2 to model 1 is 1.24 ± 2.48 mm (range, -3.28–16.41 mm). The metric can potentially be used to readily determine qualitative agreement vs disagreement using an acceptable cutoff (e.g., $<|1.5|$ mm in this figure)

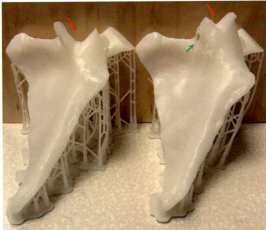 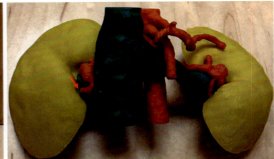

Fig. 11.3 Glenoid component models printed with bottom-up stereolithography printer (*left panel*) and bilateral renal artery aneurysms model printed with a binder jet printer (*right-hand panel*) exemplifying the need for per-model quality control procedures. A portion of the glenoid component failed to print (*red arrows*) due to large forces exerted during detachment of the model from the vat floor; additional supports (*green arrow*) enabled more of the component to successfully print but a portion still failed. Small renal artery in the binder jet model broke during removal of the model from the printer. These failures are model specific and likely would not have occurred if the models had been printed with different printer technologies; for example, the glenoid would not have failed in a binder jet system, and the renal artery would not have broken off if printed with stereolithography which uses stronger acrylic-based materials. A QC phantom printed at the same time as either of the models would have likely printed correctly, failing to capture these model-specific failures

printing technology (Fig. 11.3), for example, one that requires appropriate support structures such as SLA or FDM (see Chap. 2). The same model may print successfully using a different technology that fully surrounds the model being printed with support material, such as binder jetting, but forces exerted during cleaning of a model printed with those technologies may then lead to breakage of important anatomic features (Fig. 11.3). Visual inspection of a printed model should always be used as part of standard operating QC procedures to ensure that each finished medical model reflects the intended, segmented anatomy. Visual inspection is nonetheless prone to operator variability. The distance metric between STLs offers an alternative that is less prone to operator error. Specifically, the printed model can be scanned with CT in air, and the resulting images can be segmented to produce an STL model. This STL model can be aligned to the initial design STL that was sent to the 3D printer and the distance between the digitized model and original intended model calculated. Using,

for example, a prespecified distance cutoff that is likely to capture missing anatomy (that failed to print) can be used as a QC procedure to detect bulk errors in the printed anatomy (Fig. 11.2).

This approach does however still have limitations that render it inappropriate for many 3D printing QC procedures (George et al. 2017). One limitation is that different quantitative results are obtained depending on which model is compared to which. This is readily conceptually understood for a humeral head that has been incompletely segmented by using a HU threshold for cancellous bone (226 HU). In this example, partial volume effects in locations where the bone is thin reduce the otherwise high HU of bone, and the resulting segmentation misses the bone in those locations. The distance from points on the incomplete bone to the manually fully segmented bone is likely small, since for every point on the incomplete bone model, there is a corresponding point a short distance away on the complete model. Reversing the order of comparison, the distance from a point on the complete bone that is located in a region where the bone is missing in the incomplete model can be as far as the opposite side of the bone (Fig. 11.2). Another limitation is that digitization of a printed model introduces the point-spread function as well as modality-specific artifacts of the imaging modality, in addition to 3D printing inaccuracies. For example, in one study that imaged a printed model with both CT and MRI, each modality led to a different distance to the originally-designed STL model (Mitsouras et al. 2017). An important limitation, specific to using medical imaging modalities (as opposed to using an optical scanner) to digitize a printed model, arises from the need to segment the resulting images of the model. The resulting digitized model is highly dependent on the segmentation algorithm (George et al. 2017), even if the model is imaged in air and using an HU threshold in the range between that of air and the printed material's CT number. A study using simple cube phantoms made of materials with CT numbers equivalent to high-density bone exemplified this limitation by assessing different segmentation thresholds ranging from 25% to 95% of the difference between the HU of water (=0) and that of the material (=1400 HU). The difference between the physical phantom and its 3D-printed replica ranged from 1 mm larger to 1 mm smaller than the phantom depending on the threshold (Naitoh et al. 2006), an order of magnitude larger effect than print reproducibility. Thus, a comparison of an STL model resulting from segmentation of images of the printed model at any one given threshold will give a different result as to the distance between this digitized printed model and the original STL model sent to the printer. A final limitation of digitizing a printed model for comparison to the initially designed model is that it is necessary to align the two STL models as the scan of the printed model will inevitably use a different coordinate system reference (landmark) than the patient scan. Registration methods used for alignment, such as CloudCompare (Russ et al. 2015) or the global registration algorithm in 3-matic (Materialise NV, Belgium) CAD software are iterative optimization algorithms and may not always find a single global minimum representing the best alignment. This precludes precise comparison of the digitized model and the initially designed model toward, establishing printer QC (which would need a precision <0.5 mm in keeping with the resolution of typical clinical images), since different alignments will lead to different assessment of the distances between the models (Fig. 11.4).

11.2.2 Residual Volume

A second approach to assess the differences between STL models relies on application of mathematical set theory, considering the STL models (or segmentations) of a tissue as mathematical subsets of 3D space (George et al. 2017). In this approach, a model is intrinsically considered to define a subset of the imaged volume (i.e., of three-dimensional space) that is interpreted by the radiologist to be occupied by the tissue. Mathematical set operations can be used on these subsets to quantify differences and similarities between models. For example, agreement between two STL models can be defined by set intersection $(A \cap B)$ (George et al. 2017) (Fig. 11.5). For two models of a tissue created from interpretation of the same diagnostic images by two independent radiologists, the intersection of the two modelss simply the volume of space that both readers agreed belongs to the particular tissue. An important assembly of set intersection and union $(A \cup B)$ operations yields the so-called residual volume (Cai et al. 2015, George et al. 2017) which can be used for medical 3D printing QA. It is defined as $((A \cup B) - (A \cap B))$ (Cai et al. 2015), or, in shorthand notation as $((A\text{-}B)+(B\text{-}A))$. This is the volume occupied by one or the other model, but not both and directly quantifies the disagreement between the two models (Fig. 11.5).

These two measures of agreement and disagreement from set theory can in turn be used to define parameters commonly used to assess diagnostic accuracy, such as true and false positives and false negatives (George et al. 2017). For example, if one model is a gold standard, the true positive is the volume of space included both in

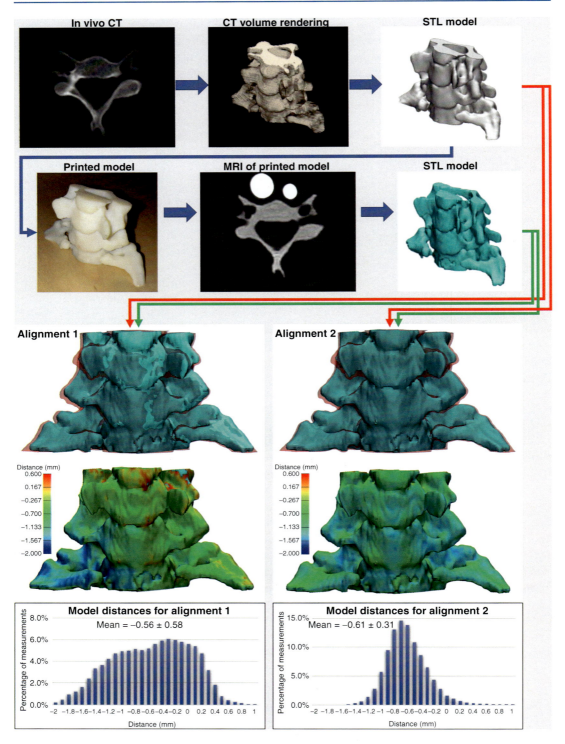

Fig. 11.4 Scanning a printed model with an imaging modality for comparison to the designed STL model should not in general be used as a QC procedure. Beyond introducing the point-spread function of the imaging modality into the errors that are being measured, model alignment algorithms are iterative optimization procedures that may converge to a local minimum, leading to different comparisons of the difference between two models

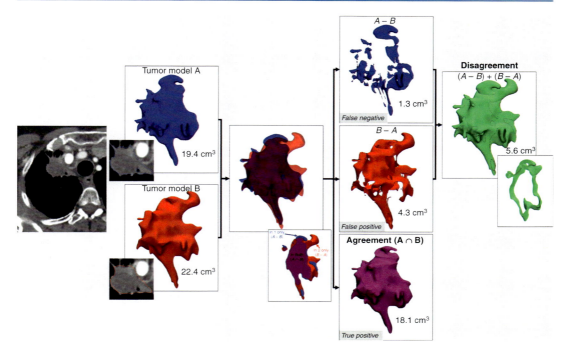

Fig. 11.5 CT of patient with superior sulcus tumor. Two qualified radiology staff members segmenting the tumor differ in their interpretation of what tissue is tumor versus what is not. The two STL models of the same tumor can be analyzed mathematically using set operations on three-dimensional space to define their disagreement and agreement. If one model is a gold standard (model A in the example shown), true positive, false negative, and false positive measures are readily calculated in terms of volume (18.1, 1.3, and 4.3 cm³, respectively). Sensitivity (true positive rate), false negative rate, and false discovery rate for the interpreter producing model B are thus readily calculated (18.1/19.4 = 93.3%, 1.3/19.4 = 6.7%, and 4.3/22.4 = 19.2%, respectively)

the test and the gold standard models, i.e., their intersection (Fig. 11.5). The volume of space included in the test model but that does not belong to the tissue according to the gold standard model, i.e., (B-A), if B is the test and A the gold standard model, is then a false positive (Fig. 11.5). Finally, the false negative volume of space is that occupied by the tissue according to the gold standard model, but that is not included in the test model (Fig. 11.5). A "true negative" volume of space is not as readily defined for general 3D printing, as it would involve the volume of space that is negative for the presence of the tissue. This could be taken to mean the entirety of a scan volume, which in most cases would be a large volume compared to that of the tissue (e.g., a single tumor seen in a chest-abdomen-pelvis CT), and would thus carry little clinical significance. However, in specific scenarios, it can be meaningfully defined, for example, for a tissue

within an organ such as a renal mass. In this case, the total kidney volume (including tumor) can be used to define the entirety of space, for which a true negative is meaningful. The volume of space within the kidney that both the test model and gold standard model agree is not tumor tissue would be the appropriate definition of the true negative volume in this example.

Using these definitions of true and false positives/negatives afforded by set theory, measures familiar to medical practitioners such as sensitivity, specificity, and accuracy can be defined for 3D-printed models whenever a gold standard (e.g., pathology findings or expert segmentation) is available. An appropriate QC program for a clinical 3D printing facility would calculate and rely on these metrics to ensure its practices enable the production of satisfactory medical models. Alternatively, agreement and disagreement between models, when neither model can be considered a gold standard, is an appropriate QA approach for a facility to compare different radiologist's interpretation in creating 3D-printed models for individual cases. Furthermore, these metrics can be used toward optimizing specific protocols for specific indications of 3D printing (George et al. 2017). An example is optimizing CT radiation dose for generating accurate models of the skull for maxillofacial surgery. Using the residual volume, we found that the increase in signal-to-noise ratio possible with iterative CT image reconstruction does not increase accuracy (i.e., does not reduce the residual volume) compared to filtered back projection. Rather, accuracy (i.e., a small residual volume) is lost equally when reducing radiation dose, regardless of the image reconstruction technique used (Cai et al. 2015).

11.3 Self-Validating Models

When the intent is to perform QC procedures on individual 3D-printed models, both mathematical measures described above encounter the limitation of alignment of the digitized model to the initial designed model. A technique that can alleviate the need for registration to assess the accuracy of a printed model was recently proposed (George et al. 2017). It involves embedding markers in a prespecified pattern (such as small spheres arranged in a unit-spaced Cartesian grid) within the printed model. The embedded marker pattern can be printed with a material of similar mechanical properties as the medical model so as to not interfere with use of the model for surgical planning, but that has different radiographic properties, for example, a different CT number. Imaging the model with the corresponding imaging modality in which the marker and model material have different image intensities would then allow assessment of dimensional accuracy by ensuring that marker spacing reflects that intended. Similarly, counting and/or matching markers to those embedded in the particular model can rapidly detect bulk anatomy missing from the printed model due to printer failure. This technique is likely to simplify printed model

QC as new printing materials that have different opacities are currently being developed.

11.4 "End-to-End" 3D Printing Quality Control

Phantom-based QC procedures can help ensure and establish the accurate, safe function of a 3D printer used to produce medical models, as well as the quality of individual medical models printed with it. It should however be noted that at present, 3D-printed phantoms should be avoided for quality control of the entire "end-to-end" process of medical 3D printing as understood to include DICOM image segmentation, STL generation, and STL post-processing. Three-dimensional-printed materials do not produce image intensities characteristic of human tissues (Mitsouras et al. 2017; Mooney et al. 2017; Shin et al. 2017; Bibb et al. 2011; Leng et al. 2016), precluding the imaging of 3D-printed models toward providing any assurances regarding the quality and accuracy of DICOM image segmentation. Furthermore, even if a QC phantom with tissue-like image intensity characteristics is used, any difference or lack thereof between the STL model obtained by segmenting will depend to some extent on the particular segmentation algorithm (e.g., the Hounsfield unit [HU] threshold) used. This is an innate limitation of all physical imaging systems, which may not have a vanishing full-width at half-maximum, complicating the assessment of model dimensions with high precision. To assess the end-to-end process of medical 3D printing, legacy (i.e., ordinarily manufactured) QC phantoms containing targets of known dimensions and different contrasts, such as the phantoms used in ACR QC procedures, should be ideally used and then only in conjunction with specific imaging protocols and specific segmentation algorithms (e.g., predetermined HU thresholds) that have been preestablished to be appropriate for segmenting each individual target using FDA-approved software for DICOM image segmentation (Di Prima et al. 2016). Such phantoms and segmentations can be the topic of future studies.

11.5 Conclusions

Quality control procedures will involve the input and research of multidisciplinary experts in the field to ensure delivery of high-quality, safe models. Physicians and medical physicists should play as strong a role as reasonable in the development of these guidelines, following the general format of those that have successfully enhanced aspects of radiology practices.

References

ACR American College of Radiology. Computed tomography quality control manual. 2012. Available from: http://www.acr.org/~/media/ACR No Index/Documents/QC Manual/2012CTQCManual1a.

ACR American College of Radiology. Magnetic Resonance Imaging Quality Control Manual. 2015. Available from: http://www.acr.org/~/media/ACR No Index/Documents/QC Manual/2015_MR_QCManual_Book.pdf.

American College of Radiology Quality & Safety. Available from: http://www.acr.org/Quality-Safety. Cited 16 April 2017.

Bibb R, Thompson D, Winder J. Computed tomography characterisation of additive manufacturing materials. Med Eng Phys. 2011;33(5):590–6.

Braian M, Jimbo R, Wennerberg A. Production tolerance of additive manufactured polymeric objects for clinical applications. Dent Mater. 2016;32(7):853–61.

Cai T, Rybicki FJ, Giannopoulos A, et al. The residual STL volume as a metric to evaluate accuracy and reproducibility of anatomic models for 3D printing: application in the validation of 3D printable models of maxillofacial bone from reduced radiation dose CT images. 3D Print Med. 2015;1(2):1–19.

Christensen A, Rybicki FJ. Maintaining safety and efficacy for 3D printing in medicine. 3D Print Med. 2017;3:1.

Di Prima M, Coburn J, Hwang D, Kelly J, Khairuzzaman A, Ricles L. Additively manufactured medical products – the FDA perspective. 3D Print Med. 2016;2(1):1.

El-Katatny I, Masood SH, Morsi YS. Error analysis of FDM fabricated medical replicas. Rapid Prototyp J. 2010;16(1):36–43.

Gelaude F, Vander Sloten J, Lauwers B. Accuracy assessment of CT-based outer surface femur meshes. Comput Aided Surg. 2008;13(4):188–99.

George E, Liacouras P, Rybicki FJ, Mitsouras D. Measuring and establishing the accuracy & reproducibility of 3D-printed medical models. Radiographics. 2017.

Leng S, Chen B, Vrieze T, et al. Construction of realistic phantoms from patient images and a commercial three-dimensional printer. J Med Imaging (Bellingham). 2016;3(3):033501.

Leng S, McGee KP, Morris JM, et al. Anatomic modeling using 3D printing: quality assurance and optimization. 3D Print Med. 2017;3:6.

Matsumoto JS, Morris JM, Foley TA, et al. Three-dimensional physical modeling: applications and experience at Mayo Clinic. Radiographics. 2015;35(7):1989–2006.

Mitsouras D, Lee TC, Liacouras P, et al. Three-dimensional printing of MRI-visible phantoms and MR image-guided therapy simulation. Magn Reson Med. 2017;77(2):613–22.

Mooney JJ, Sarwani N, Coleman ML, Fotos JS. Evaluation of three-dimensional printed materials for simulation by computed tomography and ultrasound imaging. Simul Healthc. 2017;12(3):182–8.

Naitoh M, Kubota Y, Katsumata A, Ohsaki C, Ariji E. Dimensional accuracy of a binder jet model produced from computerized tomography data for dental implants. J Oral Implantol. 2006;32(6):273–6.

Pang T, Guertin MD, Nguyen HD. Accuracy of stereolithography parts: mechanism and modes of distortion for a "Letter H" diagnostic part. In Solid freeform fabrication proceedings. 1995, p. 170.

Russ M, O'Hara R, Setlur Nagesh SV, et al. Treatment planning for image-guided neuro-vascular interventions using patient-specific 3D printed phantoms. Proc SPIE Int Soc Opt Eng. 2015;9417:11.

Salmi M, Paloheimo KS, Tuomi J, Wolff J, Makitie A. Accuracy of medical models made by additive manufacturing (rapid manufacturing). J Craniomaxillofac Surg. 2013;41(7):603–9.

Shin J, Sandhu RS, Shih G. Imaging properties of 3D printed materials: multi-energy CT of filament polymers. J Digit Imaging 2017 Feb 6. doi:10.1007/s10278-017-9954-9 [Epub ahead of print].

Teeter MG, Kopacz AJ, Nikolov HN, Holdsworth DW. Metrology test object for dimensional verification in additive manufacturing of metals for biomedical applications. Proceedings of the institution of mechanical engineers, part H. J Eng Med. 2015;229(1):20–7.

U.S. Food and Drug Administration. Technical considerations for additive manufactured devices: draft guidance for industry and food and drug administration staff. 2016. Available from: https://www.fda.gov/downloads/MedicalDevices/DeviceRegulationandGuidance/GuidanceDocuments/UCM499809.pdf. Cited 2016.

Wake N, Rude T, Kang SK, et al. 3D printed renal cancer models derived from MRI data: application in pre-surgical planning. Abdom Radiol (NY). 2017;42(5):1501–9.

Weinstock P, Prabhu SP, Flynn K, Orbach DB, Smith E. Optimizing cerebrovascular surgical and endovascular procedures in children via personalized 3D printing. J Neurosurg Pediatr. 2015:1–6 [Epub ahead of print].

Virtual Reality

12

Justin Sutherland and Dan La Russa

12.1 Introduction

Recent technological advances have increased the quality and accessibility of compelling, immersive virtual reality (VR) (Largent 2011), motivating its wider adoption in the domain of radiology and medicine in general. The ability to effectively and flexibly visualize segmented medical models as well as unsegmented image data makes virtual reality an attractive modality to complement a medical 3D printing program. This chapter presents an overview of virtual reality and its history, describes the current landscape of modern VR technology, and describes current and future medical applications including its relationship to 3D printing.

J. Sutherland, Ph.D., M.C.C.P.M. (✉)
Radiation Medicine Program, Department of Medical Physics, The Ottawa Hospital, Ottawa, ON, Canada

Cancer Therapeutics Program, Ottawa Hospital Research Institute, Ottawa, ON, Canada
e-mail: jussutherland@toh.ca

D. La Russa, Ph.D., F.C.C.P.M.
Radiation Medicine Program, Department of Medical Physics, The Ottawa Hospital, Ottawa, ON, Canada

Cancer Therapeutics Program, Ottawa Hospital Research Institute, Ottawa, ON, Canada

Division of Medical Physics, Department of Radiology, University of Ottawa,
Ottawa, ON, Canada
e-mail: dlarussa@toh.ca

Virtual reality has been broadly defined as "a high-end user-computer interface that involves real-time simulation and interactions through multiple sensorial channels" (Largent 2011). Two hallmarks of virtual reality are visualization and positional tracking. The real-time visualization required for virtual reality has historically been achieved primarily through head-mounted devices (HMDs) that use small screens and lenses to cover the user's visual field or CAVE Automatic Virtual Environments (CAVEs) that take the form of cube-like spaces in which images are displayed by a series of projectors (Burdea and Coiffet 2003). To relate the visual information being displayed to the user to a simulated virtual environment, the position of the user's eyes (or head) must be tracked in 3D space. Full positional (six degrees of freedom) or rotational-only (three degrees of freedom) tracking have commonly been accomplished through the use of inertial monitor units (IMUs) (Burdea and Coiffet 2003), computer vision (Foxlin et al. 1998), laser-based tracking (SteamVR® Tracking 2017), magnetic tracking (Burdea and Coiffet 2003), or a combination of these technologies.

The terms virtual, augmented, or mixed reality have recently become buzzwords following the growing popularity of new consumer VR devices. These sometimes confusing terms are clearly explained and delineated by the concept of the reality-virtuality continuum first introduced by Milgram et al. (1994) and illustrated in Fig. 12.1. On one end of the continuum, there are

© Springer International Publishing AG 2017
F.J. Rybicki, G.T. Grant (eds.), *3D Printing in Medicine*, DOI 10.1007/978-3-319-61924-8_12

Fig. 12.1 Illustration of the reality-virtuality continuum

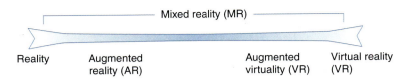

environments consisting entirely of the real world: reality. On the other, environments that consist entirely of virtual objects: virtual reality (VR). Mixed reality (MR), then, is defined as a continuum between the two extremes where there is some combination of real and virtual environments—augmented reality (AR) being a subset. Augmented reality describes a simulation where the majority of the environment experienced is that of the real world, but with some amount of added virtual objects or environments. The less common concept of augmented virtuality (AV) describes a fully immersive virtual environment that has added elements of the real world (by using live video input, for example).

12.2 History of Virtual Reality

12.2.1 Early Milestones

While the concept of VR dates back to early science fiction writers, its history is rooted in the idea of an "experience theater," described by Morton Heilig around 1950 (Burdea and Coiffet 2003). The focus of Heilig's idea was a cinematic experience for users involving all the senses rather than just the usual 2D display with sound. Twelve years later, in 1962, Heilig introduced the Sensorama Simulator (US Patent # 3,050,870): an arcade-style device for a single user that featured displays of 3D video feedback (obtained by a pair of side-by-side 35 mm cameras), stereo sound, a moving chair, wind effects via small fans near the user's head, and even odor producers. The Sensorama is considered the earliest archetype of immersive, multisensory technologies.

Heilig may also be the first to propose head-worn displays with his concept of a simulation mask. He was granted a patent for his concept in 1960 (US Patent # 2,955,156), which featured 3D analog displays encompassing the user's periph-

ery, optical controls, stereophonic sound, and smells. In 1961, Philco Corporation introduced their version of a headset device tethered to a closed-circuit television system that could be used by the wearer to transmit findings while navigating dangerous environments. However, it was Ivan Sutherland who is credited with producing the first example of a fully immersive head-mounted display (HMD; sometimes called the head-mounted audio-visual display). Released in 1966, and called the *Sword of Damocles*, Sutherland's HMD used two cathode ray tubes to produce a stereoscopic display with a 40° field of view. The device was suspended from a ceiling-mounted cantilever—being too heavy to be supported by the wearer—which also tracked the wearer's viewing direction via potentiometers. Sutherland later incorporated computer-generated scenes to take the place of analog images with his groundbreaking development of a scene generator that produced primitive 3D wireframe graphics. Introduced in 1973, Sutherland's scene generator was capable of displaying 200–400 polygons per scene (frame) at a rate of 20 frames per second. These scene generators are the precursors to modern graphics accelerators—a key component of VR computer hardware.

Other important elements of immersive experiences followed shortly after the emergence of HMDs. In 1971, the first example of haptic feedback was demonstrated by Frederick Brooks Jr. and his colleagues. This development, as well as others, was incorporated into several iterations of military flight simulations in the 1970s and 1980s which was classified at the time. Other government agencies were also pursuing their own interests in simulators. In 1981, the National Aeronautics and Space Agency (NASA) created an HMD that used liquid crystal displays with optical controls to focus the images they produced close to the eyes. The initial NASA device was called the Virtual Visual Environment Display, or VIVED. Their successor system, called the VIEW for Virtual Interface Environment Workstation, was introduced in the late 1980s and boasted upgraded computer hardware as well as an interactive glove for manipulating wireframe objects that were spatially and mechanically tracked.

By the late 1980s and early 1990s, commercial VR systems began to emerge. The DataGlove, the same glove used by NASA's VIEW system, was introduced in 1987 by VPL Inc. and was the first break from the standard keyboard and mouse computer interface tools. VPL Inc. was also the first company to release an immersive VR solution consisting of an HMD (called, interestingly, the *EyePhone*) that featured two LCD displays to produce stereoscopic images, each with a resolution of just 360 × 240 pixels. The HMD was used together with their previously released DataGlove, and their system was called the RB2 system (Reality Built for 2). It retailed for over $11,000.00, and the HMD weighed over 5 lbs. Nintendo later released an answer to the DataGlove in 1993, called the Power Glove.

While hand-worn and head-mounted devices were under development, other companies focused on improving VR hardware and software platforms. In 1991, Division Ltd. in the UK produced a scalable and integrated VR workstation to support their line of VR products. On the software side, the US company Sense8 in 1992 developed a library of VR-specific programming functions, called the WorldToolKit. This was followed by the Virtual Reality Toolkit (VRT3) software framework by Dimensions International in the UK.

12.2.2 Alternative Technological Approaches

While head-worn displays are currently considered the de facto standard for fully immersive VR and are the most practical technological solution for consumers, previous limitations associated with HMDs (e.g., weight) motivated the exploration of other VR system concepts. One popular example is the cave automatic virtual environment (CAVE) or its variations. A CAVE is a small room enclosed by whole-wall displays of virtual images produced by a series of video projectors.

A stereoscopic 3D effect can be achieved through the use of positionally tracked active shutter glasses worn by the occupants and synced with the projectors. In active shuttering, the projected image alternates between the views for the left and right eye, while a shutter blocks the eye for which the view does not apply, producing a 3D perspective. CAVEs are commonly used in engineering, manufacturing, and construction industries to prototype designs.

12.2.3 Historical Applications in Medicine

The earliest applications of VR in medicine were centered around visualizing medical images and performing surgical planning (Chinnock 1994). Since then, medical applications of VR have expanded into the realm of medical education and training, facilitated communication (between clinicians or between clinicians and patients), and in a variety of therapies, including the treatment of phobias, PTSD, anxiety disorders, rehabilitation, and pain management. Interest in medical applications of VR has also been steadily accumulating. A recent search by Pensieri and Pennacchini (2014), for VR-related articles in the medical literature, uncovered nearly 12,000 publications as of 2012 using the most common search terms representative of VR applications in healthcare (but excluding "virtual environment," "augmented reality," etc.). Rather than focusing on the traditional applications of VR in medicine, the rest of this chapter will focus on the current landscape of VR technologies and how these technologies may be used to enhance the domain of 3D printing and the domain of 3D visualization in general.

12.2.4 A Technology Outpaced by Vision

Despite the pace of early development, as well as considerable amounts of media attention, VR companies in the 1990s failed to secure a widespread consumer base. Early systems were prohibitively expensive, with the fastest available graphics workstation by Silicon Graphics Inc. costing over $100,000, and were plagued with performance and reliability issues. As such, the VR industry remained small and largely contained to corporations, government institutions, and universities despite several attempts by the video game industry to generate interest in VR systems. Eventually, the rise of the internet claimed the public's attention and, subsequently, interest in VR technologies waned when the few remaining companies failed to deliver on media hype (Stone 2006).

12.3 Modern Commercial Virtual Reality Technologies

12.3.1 Renewed Interest in VR

A new era of affordable virtual reality technology has recently emerged—driven primarily by the video game industry and enabled by breakthroughs in smartphone display technology, graphic processing units (GPUs), and tracking technology. VR recaptured significant public attention in 2012 largely due to the successful crowd-funding campaign for the Oculus Rift (Oculus VR, Menlo Park, CA) (Largent 2011; Kickstarter 2012). The campaign presented a prototype of a rotationally-tracked HMD using IMUs and smartphone displays. Following two developer kits and acquisition of Oculus by Facebook (Largent 2011), the Oculus Rift consumer version was released in March of 2016—consisting of a high-resolution, low latency head-mounted display. Six degrees of freedom positional tracking of the HMD is facilitated by a proprietary tracking system called Constellation which uses IMUs and optical cameras that track infrared (IR), patterned LED markers. Tracked handheld controllers were later released for the Rift in December of 2016.

While Oculus received the bulk of public attention throughout its development of the Rift, the emergence of modern VR technology resulted from the work of a number of players. One notable example is Valve Corporation (Bellevue, WA) who are credited with the development or discovery of a number of key components that facilitate immersive VR (e.g., the necessity of low-

persistence displays) (James 2015). Following an early collaborative relationship with Oculus, Valve partnered with HTC Corporation (New Taipei City, China) to produce the HTC Vive—released 1 month after the Oculus Rift. The Vive was released with tracked controllers and uses a full room-scale, 360° tracking system called SteamVR® Tracking. SteamVR Tracking uses IMUs in conjunction with two "base stations" that regularly sweep the room with IR lasers (which are detected by photodiodes on the tracked objects) and boasts high-frequency sub-millimeter tracking accuracy within a 5 m corner-to-corner volume (SteamVR® Tracking 2017).

Together, the Oculus Rift and HTC Vive represent the first widely available, modern, PC-based, consumer VR platforms. However, the new landscape of VR devices is rapidly evolving with other offerings such as Razer OSVR, FOVE, MindMaze MindLeap, and Vrvana Totem which all present interesting technological variations (Largent 2011). With many choices available, and certainly more to come, early adopters of modern VR will likely be concerned with compatibility both now and in the future. To this end, Valve has made their SteamVR® software platform open to all hardware manufacturers through the OpenVR software development kit and application programming interface and have even gone so far as to freely license the use of SteamVR® Tracking so that any hardware manufacturer can make use of their tracking system (SteamVR® Tracking 2017; Lee 2017). The future of VR technology compatibility will also likely be greatly facilitated by the development of OpenXR: a cross-platform open standard for virtual reality and augmented reality applications and devices created in collaboration with a group of companies under the direction of the Khronos Group (Khronos Group 2017).

12.3.2 Mobile VR

Beyond advances in PC-based or "tethered" virtual reality technology, modern developments have also introduced a new domain of *mobile* VR driven primarily by smartphones. These devices take the form of custom lenses mounted in cases of various designs that hold compatible smartphones. Software is run on the smartphones themselves, and tracking—accomplished by relying on the phone's internal IMUs or mounted IMUs—is generally limited to rotational (three degrees of freedom) only. Current examples of mobile VR at the time of writing are the Samsung Gear VR (Samsung, Seoul, South Korea), Google Cardboard (Google, Mountain View, CA) (simply a handheld cardboard shell with lenses), and Google Daydream (Wiederhold 2016).

Considering that the computational ability of smartphones is significantly less than that of high-end PCs and that mobile VR is generally limited to rotational-only tracking, the experiences available with mobile VR have been comparatively limited in capability to date. Despite this, mobile VR has already been used in medical roles such as anatomical education (Moro et al. 2017), ophthalmic image display (Zheng et al. 2015), surgical training (Gallagher et al. 2016), and patient education (Forani 2017).

With various classes of VR experiences available—from simpler mobile experiences to high-end PC experiences with external tracking systems—it is useful to distinguish between different levels of HMD-based VR experiences by the sophistication of their visualization and tracking. The most basic, perhaps, are 360° videos. These experiences are created from video recordings where a view in every direction is simultaneously recorded using an omnidirectional camera or a collection of cameras. The VR user then controls viewing direction with rotational-only head tracking (Forani 2017), and since the video is monoscopic and parallax is impossible, there is no perception of depth by the user. With more sophisticated video recording technology, 360° videos can be recorded with stereoscopic cameras adding the perception of depth to the video viewing experience. However, translation of head position is not reflected in the experience and interaction with the environment is not possible.

When the position and orientation of the user's head is tracked in 3D space, the convincing sensation of being present in a fully immersive virtual space can be realized. However, this precludes the use of prerecorded video, and virtual experiences must now be generated in real time

by a 3D rendering engine. Including tracked hand or controller positions increases the level of interaction available and creates an even more immersive experience (Cameron et al. 2011).

12.3.3 Augmented Reality

The new enthusiasm for virtual reality has also increased the attention given to augmented reality. This technology has recently taken the form of handheld experiences using smartphones and tablets where digital models are superimposed onto the real world (Moro et al. 2017); video pass-through headsets where forward mounted cameras are placed on the front of virtual reality headsets and stereoscopic video of the real world is superimposed with virtual images (Largent 2011; VRVana 2017; uSens Inc. 2016; Abrash 2012); and see-through glasses—most notably illustrated by the Microsoft Hololens development kit (Microsoft® 2017)—where virtual elements are superimposed on clear glasses or visors with additive blending (Largent 2011, Abrash 2012).

While augmented reality technology holds great promise for medical practitioners, and current solutions are being used by some groups (Cui et al. 2017; Weng and Bee 2016; Garon 2016), the communication from leaders in the field suggests it may be several years before augmented reality headsets see widespread proliferation (Brennan 2017). This is largely due to the current limitations and greater challenges that the technology faces compared to virtual reality.

For video pass-through AR, the experience is diminished by the fact that video has a lower dynamic range and resolution than real-world vision. Additionally, the eye is not free to focus on any part of the real world since focus is controlled by the cameras. The need to overcome latency introduced by capture, processing, and display of the real-world images can also be a challenge (Abrash 2012).

The challenges concerning perceiving the real world are bypassed in see-through AR methods where the real world is simply viewed directly.

However, tracking for see-through headsets is generally accomplished through inside-out, computer vision solutions which introduce some latency, especially for mobile form factors. Since there is no delay associated with visualizing the real world, small lag in the positioning and visualization of virtual elements—which often must interact with real-world objects—is more easily noticed. See-through AR also faces the challenge of only being able to display virtual elements through additive blending, which means that visualization is necessarily translucent and pure black cannot be generated (Abrash 2012). Finally, current implementations of see-through display technology result in small fields-of-view for virtual element visualization, resulting in a limited ability to blend virtual elements with the real world in a convincing manner (Ren et al. 2016; Kreylos 2015).

12.4   Medical Virtual Reality and 3D Printing

Due to new levels of robust performance, accessibility, and low cost, the emerging ecosystem of modern virtual and augmented reality technologies promises to revolutionize the practice of medicine in ways that previous technological iterations did not. Modern computer graphics hardware allows for the real-time, fluid visualization of computationally intense medical data. New, cost-effective, and robust tracking systems open the door for intuitive human interactions with virtual medical models. Finally, advances in computer vision and holographic visualization technologies increase the accessibility of mixed reality tools for facilitating medical interventions.

While virtual reality has a rich history of being researched (see Sect. 12.2.3), until recently, medical VR applications have seen relatively limited clinical adoption. However, there is currently a booming interest in many different medical uses of VR. For example, the domain of medical training and education has seen a recent increase in publications (Matzke

et al. 2017; Zilverschoon et al. 2017; Rahm et al. 2016; Hackett and Sttc 2013; Herron 2016). Much of what makes 3D printing attractive as a teaching tool can be applied to the visualization of medical models in virtual reality. What VR visualization methods lack in their inability to be interacted with as physical objects, they make up for in flexibility: animation, varying transparency, resizing, movable cut planes, etc. are all possible with the same sense of depth and 3D understanding that comes with handling 3D-printed models.

Virtual reality is also likely to make a significant impact on patient education. It has already been used to alleviate patient anxiety toward medical procedures (Forani 2017) and can be used, much like 3D-printed models, to explain pathology and medical details to patients (MediVis 2017).

Due to its ability to flexibly simulate the medical data related to patients or immerse clinicians in a realistic environment, there is a renewed interest in using virtual and augmented reality to improve surgery and surgical planning. Several systems for surgical training are currently available or in development (Osso VR 2017; BioflightVR 2017; 3D Systems 2017), and several systems for augmented reality-guided interventions are being researched or used (RealView Imaging Ltd. 2017; Baum et al. 2017) with many more likely to emerge in the coming years.

Of particular interest to adopters of medical 3D printing is perhaps the use of VR for medical image visualization (MediVis 2017; Surgical Theater LLC 2017; Cattin 2016; EchoPixel 2017; Vizua Inc. 2017). In contrast with 3D printing, virtual reality can be used to visualize unsegmented image sets through volume rendering (Zhang et al. 2011). Applying volume rendering techniques in VR is likely to be an active area of research in computer science since the computational requirements (two images for stereoscopy, high frame rate requirement, high resolution) for virtual reality increase the demands on what is already a relatively high computational load. More sophisticated volume rendering techniques

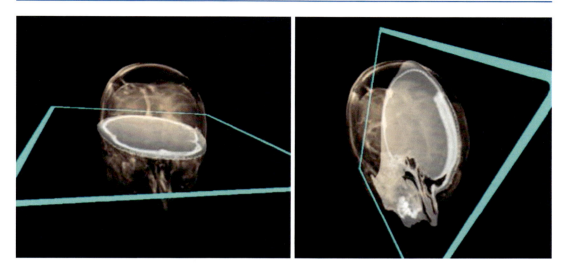

Fig. 12.2 Example of interacting with volume rendering image sets (fused MRI and CT) using a handheld virtual plane to navigate through the image set in any arbitrary orientation

(Dappa et al. 2016) will likely require modification or optimization before they can perform at a high enough frame rate for fully immersive VR. In addition to the realistic perception of depth and scale that virtual reality provides, the use of handheld tracked controllers allows for intuitive manipulation of medical images as illustrated in Fig. 12.2, which shows the use of a handheld visualization plane being used to interact with a CT-MRI fusion.

VR can also be used to visualize segmented medical models. The STL or other object files generated for 3D printing take little to no effort to import into accessible 3D rendering engines such as Unity (Unity Technologies, San Francisco, CA) or Unreal Engine (Epic Games, Cary, NC). With VR system plugins for these engines being freely available, there is very little overhead for developing simple medical VR applications for research or clinical use. The flexibility that virtual reality provides when interacting with 3D models provides a useful parallel avenue to 3D printing for the clinical use of medical models (see illustration in Fig. 12.3), and a wide range of innovative and impactful VR applications will likely develop from this new creative space.

Virtual reality may well become a facilitator for future medical 3D printing practices.

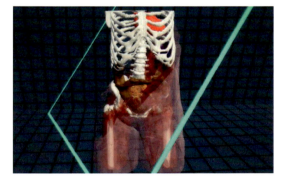

Fig. 12.3 Example of interacting with medical models in virtual reality illustrating the benefit of controllable variations in transparency

Recent software developments outside the medical domain have already shown a diverse number of examples of VR effectively facilitating sculpting and modeling (Oculus VR LLC 2017; MakeVR 2017; Brinx Software 2016) with the resulting models often being physically realized with 3D printing (MakeVR 2017; Brinx Software 2016; Strange 2017). It is easy to imagine that with the ability to effectively visualize 3D scan sets and intuitively manipulate 3D models, the medical model creation workflow could be greatly enhanced by virtual reality.

12.5　Conclusions

Previous iterations of virtual reality technology suffered from premature enthusiasm and mostly failed to live up to expectations. However, a recent confluence of technological innovations has led to a new environment of rapid development and growing adoption which suggests that, this time, VR is here to stay. Forward-thinking medical professionals would do well to pay close attention to what promises to be both a strong complement to 3D printing and a transformative technology in its own right.

References

3D Systems. 2017. https://www.3dsystems.com.

Abrash M. 2012. http://blogs.valvesoftware.com/abrash/why-you-wont-see-hard-ar-anytimesoon/.

Baum Z, Ungi T, Lasso A, Fichtinger G. Usability of a real-time tracked augmented reality display system in musculoskeletal injections. In SPIE medical imaging 2017: image-guided procedures, robotic interventions, and modeling, 2017.

BioflightVR. 2017. http://www.immersus.co/.

Garon M, Boulet PO, Doironz JP, Beaulieu L, Lalonde JF. Real-time High Resolution 3D Data on the HoloLens. 2016 IEEE International Symposium on Mixed and Augmented Reality (ISMAR-Adjunct), 2016. p. 189–91

Brennan D. 2017. http://www.roadtovr.com/oculus-chief-scientist-michael-abrash-exploresaugmented-reality-future-f8-facebook/.

Brinx Software. 2016. http://brinxvr.com/mpvr.

Burdea GC, Coiffet P. Virtual reality technology. 2nd ed. New York: John Wiley & Sons, Inc.; 2003.

Cameron CR, DiValentin LW, Manaktala R, McElhaney AC, Nostrand CH, Quinlan OJ, Sharpe LN, Slagle AC, Wood CD, Zheng YY, Gerling GJ. Hand tracking and visualization in a virtual reality simulation. In 2011 IEEE systems and information engineering design symposium, vol 22904, 2011. p. 127–32.

Cattin PC. 2016. https://www.unibas.ch/en/News-Events/News/Uni-Research/Virtual-Reality-in-Medicine.html.

Chinnock C. Virtual reality in surgery and medicine. Hosp Technol Ser. 1994;13:1–48.

Cui N, Kharel P, Gruev V. Augmented reality with Microsoft HoloLens holograms for near infrared fluorescence based image guided surgery. Proc SPIE. 2017;10049:1–6.

Dappa E, Higashigaito K, Fornaro J, Leschka S, Wildermuth S, Alkadhi H. Cinematic rendering – an alternative to volume rendering for 3D computed tomography imaging. Insights Imaging. 2016;7:849–56.

EchoPixel. 2017. http://www.echopixeltech.com.

Forani J. 2017. https://www.thestar.com/life/health_wellness/2017/03/20/toronto-hospitalsembrace-virtual-reality.html.

Foxlin E, Harrington M, Pfeifer G. Constellation: a wide-range wireless motion tracking system for augmented reality and virtual set applications. In Proceedings of the 25th annual conference on computer graphics and interactive techniques—SIGGRAPH '98, 98, 1998. p. 371–8.

Gallagher K, Jain S, Okhravi N. Making and viewing stereoscopic surgical videos with smartphones and virtual reality headset. Eye. 2016;30:503–4.

Hackett M, Sttc A-h. Medical holography for basic anatomy training medical holography for basic anatomy training, 2013. p. 1–10.

Herron J. Augmented reality in medical education and training. J Electr Resour Med Librar. 2016;13:51–5.

James P. 2015. http://www.roadtovr.com/valve-reveals-timeline-of-vive-prototypes-we-chart-it-for-you.

Khronos Group. 2017. https://www.khronos.org/openxr/.

Kickstarter. 2012. https://www.kickstarter.com/projects/1523379957/oculus-rift-step-into-the-game.

Kreylos O. HoloLens and field of view in augmented reality. 2015. http://doc-ok.org/?p=1274.

Largent D. Crossroads the ACM magazine for students. 2011. Xrds.Acm.Org.

Lee N. 2017. https://www.engadget.com/2017/03/02/lg-steamvr-headset/.

MakeVR. 2017. http://www.viveformakers.com/.

Matzke J, Ziegler C, Martin K, Crawford S, Sutton E. Usefulness of virtual reality in assessment of medical student laparoscopic skill. J Surg Res. 2017;211: 191–5.

MediVis. 2017. http://www.mediv.is/.

Microsoft®. 2017. https://www.microsoft.com/en-us/hololens.

Milgram P, Takemura H, Utsumi A, Kishino F. Mixed reality (MR) reality-virtuality (RV) continuum. Syst Res. 1994;2351:282–92.

Moro C, Štromberga Z, Raikos A, Stirling A. The effectiveness of virtual and augmented reality in health sciences and medical anatomy. AnatSci Educ. 2017.

Oculus VR LLC. 2017. https://www.oculus.com/medium/.

Osso VR. 2017. http://ossovr.com/.

Pensieri C, Pennacchini M. Overview: virtual reality in medicine. J Virtual Worlds Res. 2014;7:1–34.

Rahm S, Wieser K, Wicki I, Holenstein L, Fucentese SF, Gerber C. Performance of medical students on a virtual reality simulator for knee arthroscopy: an analysis of learning curves and predictors of performance. BMC Surg. 2016;16:1–8.

RealView Imaging Ltd. 2017. http://realviewimaging.com.

Ren D, Goldschwendt T, Chang Y, Hollerer T. Evaluating wide-field-of-view augmented reality with mixed reality simulation. In proceedings – IEEE virtual reality, July 2016. p. 93–102.

uSens Inc.. 2016. https://usens.com/.

SteamVR® Tracking. 2017. https://partner.steamgames.com/vrtracking.

Stone RJ. Virtual reality: virtual and synthetic environments - technologies and applications. Boca Raton, FL: Taylor & Francis Group LLC; 2006.

Strange A. 2017. http://mashable.com/2017/01/19/oculus-medium-sculpture/.

Surgical Theater LLC. 2017. www.surgicaltheater.net.

Vizua Inc.. 2017. https://vizua3d.com.

Vrvana. 2017. https://vrvana.com/.

Weng NG, Bee OY. An augmented reality system for biology science education in Malaysia. Int J Innov Comput. 2016;6:8–13.

Wiederhold BK. Annual review of CyberTherapy and telemedicine. Being different: the transformative potential, Interactive Media Institute, vol. 14. San Diego, CA; 2016.

Zhang Q, Eagleson R, Peters TM. Volume visualization: a technical overview with a focus on medical applications. J Digit Imaging. 2011;24:640–64.

Zheng LL, He L, Yu CQ. Mobile virtual reality for ophthalmic image display and diagnosis. J Mob Technol Med. 2015;4:35–8.

Zilverschoon M, Vincken KL, Bleys RLAW. The virtual dissecting room: creating highly detailed anatomy models for educational purposes. J Biomed Inform. 2017;65:58–75.

Index

© Springer International Publishing AG 2017
F.J. Rybicki, G.T. Grant (eds.), *3D Printing in Medicine*, DOI 10.1007/978-3-319-61924-8